Sweetness and Light

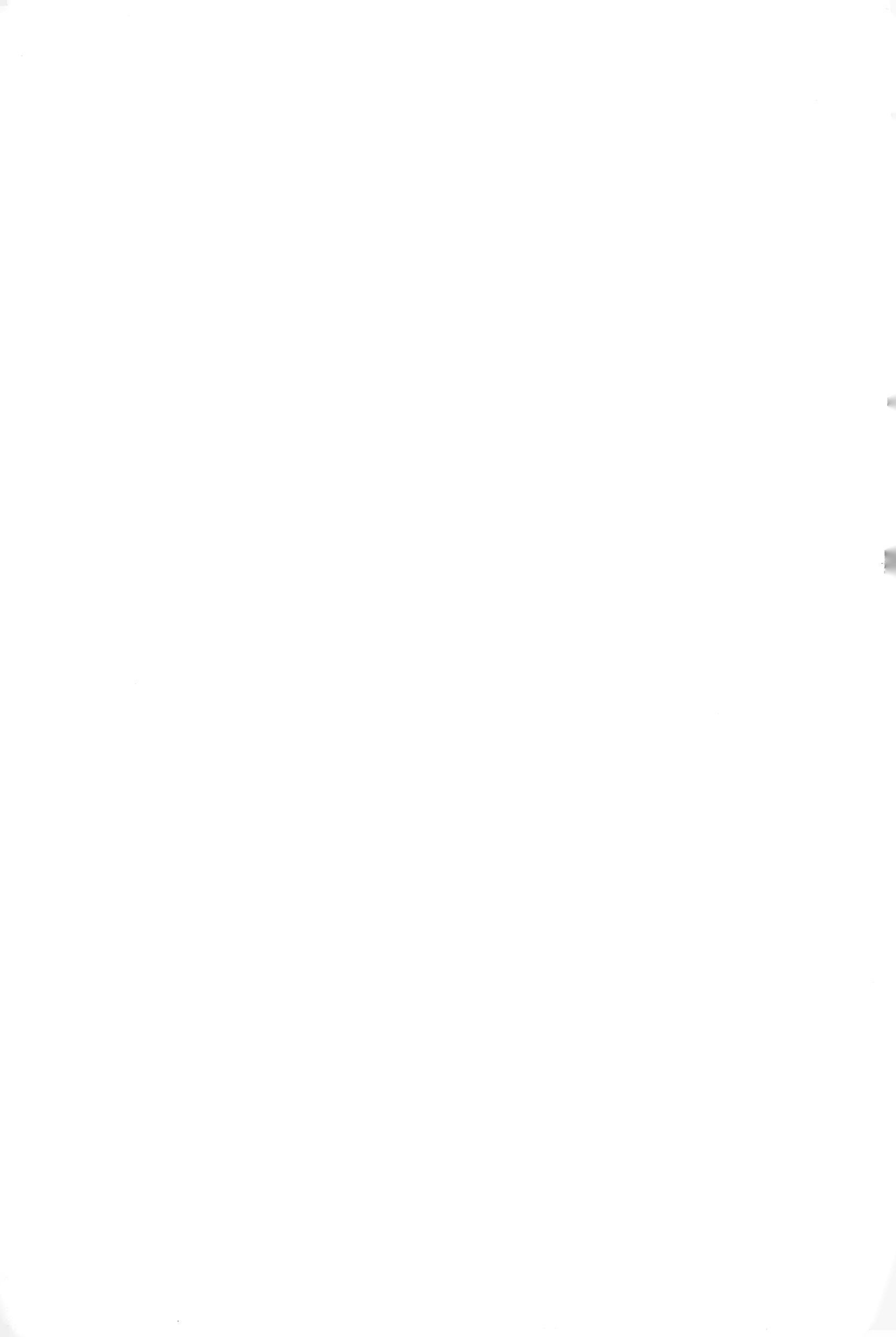

Christopher Emsden

Sweetness and Light

Why the demonization of sugar does not make sense

McGraw-Hill Education

Milano • New York • Bogotá • Lisbon • London
Madrid • Mexico City • Montreal • New Delhi
Santiago • Seoul • Singapore • Sydney • Toronto

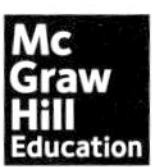

McGraw-Hill Education (Italy) S.r.l.
via Ripamonti 89, 20141 Milano

Programme and Portfolio Manager: Natalie Jacobs
Programme Manager: Marta Colnago
Acquisition Editor: Daniele Bonanno
Production: Donatella Giuliani
Typesetting: Eicon, Torino
Editing: Jonathan Ingoldby, Publishing Services, Brighton
Cover Design: Jonathan Bargus
Cover Image: © iStock.com/George Clerk
Stampa: KINT, Ljubljana, Slovenia

ISBN 978-88-386-7495-2
Printed in Slovenia

Table of Contents

Foreword

Sugar is generally associated with something positive, desirable and indeed sweet. In recent years, however, sugar has been suggested as one of the major factors contributing to diabetes and obesity epidemics. A number of scientific studies report associations between the amount of sugar eaten and the Body Mass Index (BMI), the most common method to measure overweight and obesity. Results of these studies are straightforward: the higher the consumption of sugar the higher the BMI. There is indeed very little doubt that people who are overweight and obese generally eat too much sugar in all the forms it is available in our daily life. The point, however, is that they are likely to eat too much of everything.

By many scientific and policy-driven quarters, it is suggested that eating sugar is unhealthy and thus that interventions need to be designed to help people to reduce its consumption. While this book does not take an open standing against the aim of reducing sugar consumption, he tries to broaden the perspective from which we look at nutrition. The book uses scientific sources from both the biomedical and the social sciences to make readers thinking beyond the common and standard way used to look at nutrition behaviour and policies. Through reference to scientific papers, reporting opinions of experts and persuasive argumentations Mr Emsden challenges a number of common wisdoms about eating sugar, its risk for human health and policies aimed at reducing its consumption.

The book is too rich of examples, cases and ideas to be summarised and, in my view, its main contribution to the extant literature is to make people thinking harder than it is often the case. Being a Policy Analysis person, reading the book has made me thinking harder on a number of themes with policy implications.

Obesity is not simply a new disease deserving well-focused prevention measures and even major medical treatments, such as surgery to reduce the length of the gut. Obesity, more than other unhealthy conditions, is the outcome of a number of genetic, biological, social, economic and cultural factors that cannot be ignored by both the scientific community and policy makers. For the author obesity is also a social construction that is shaped by the way is measured, reported to the public and made important by the scientific community. The author takes the reader through several examples which show how social institutions shape the "obese" and the way is treated (medically and socially).

Mr Emsden, a well-known journalist with a deep understanding of both biological and social sciences, is also ready to discuss the role of evidence even from a more positivist attitude towards science. He highlights the interactions between the environment, both social and natural, and eating behaviour. These interactions are very complex and still mostly unknown and under-investigated. But the little already known suggests that poverty, social marginalisation, unemployment, job insecurity are all important factors that create the humus for several unhealthy and "self-inflicted" conditions including obesity. Thus, very specific measures that address specific nutrients are likely to have little impact because they address just the symptom (over-nutrition and malnutrition) of a general human condition that is the real and deep cause of ill-health. In addition, too much emphasis on very specific risk factors and narrow interventions may obscure the general picture that it is indeed one of increasing inequalities and emerging forms of human deprivation. In that, he suggests some evocative expressions to expand our view of nutrition and its determinants. My favourite is "metabolic ghettos": physical, psychological and even physiological ghettos where people do not only face "food deserts", that is lack of healthy food in the surroundings, but are also without the basic capabilities to properly manage their life, including nutritional choices.

The frequent reference to the scientific literature about nutrition has made me thinking about the type of science we need to fight morbidity and mortality attributable to poor diets. Most of the literature cited in the book is bio-medical and reports quantitative studies which try prove or falsify hypotheses about cause-effects relations.

However, my understanding is that this literature, and that used to support a number of polices in the field of nutrition, is mainly showing correlations; it suggests association between variables but very often does not provide evidence of causation. Think again at "food deserts", which are the areas mainly located in the US where only low-quality and junk food is available. Living in these areas is clearly associated to obesity and ill health . But this association does not imply causation and, more importantly, does not imply that just providing more opportunities of healthier food may have a positive impact on its consumption. Food deserts result from a number of socio-economic factors and it may be difficult to disentangle their direct effects from those of the underlying societal conditions. People may find vendors of healthy food in the surrounding but may decide not to buy anything there for a number of reasons, including the higher prices of most of healthy food. In other words, are people obese because they cannot find good quality food in their neighborough or because they live in poor, deprived, marginalised, violent communities that make people's coping with life harder? It might be the very case that pouring money to improve a bit the supply of healthy food in those communities has no effect because does not address the real factors determining behavioural and social choices leading to poor nutrition and ill health.

The book has made me thinking at two additional major issues about the role of science in nutrition. The first concerns the standard of evidence about the effects of nutrition on health. We know very well the standards required by regulatory agencies for pharmaceuticals in the US and Europe. These standards are very demanding, although it is often suggested that they should be even stricter. They require large investments in research and development with high risk of failure. The high prices of pharmaceuticals and the extra-profits that pharmaceutical companies reap are also due to these stringent criteria used by policy makers. Compared to these standard, those in nutrition appears very modest. The recent evidence on the risk of cardio-vascular diseases attributable to animal and vegetal fats is an alarming example in this respect. Likely, the evidence used by policy makers in the past was very weak by any scientific standard.

Actually, I remember the campaigns to use (hydrogenated) margarine to replace butter in the 1970s. Now we all know that the promotion of margarine at that time was a mistake. Bad science or bad use of modest scientific evidence drove unhealthy and costly choices.

Running randomized clinical trials is very expensive and often poses major ethical problems. This is likely to be even more so in the nutrition field. Not surprisingly very few randomized trials on nutrition are thus conducted and, as a result, the quality of evidence to offer guidance to food and nutrition policies for their impact on health is poor and can be easily manipulated by vested interests of different kinds, from those of the industry to those in need to justify new taxes. Unfortunately, the brutal true is that without better evidence about nutrition policies the risk to design ineffective, costly and even unpopular policies is very high.

High quality evidence from randomized trials or well conducted quasi-experiments is essential to understand whether and how we should alter our nutrition behaviour. I suspect that this evidence, in addition to be difficult to produce, presents "generalization" problems more relevant than those for drugs and medical technologies given the interactions between nutrition, the social and the natural environment. This is because it looks unlikely that the desirable quantity of a specific nutrient be independent of ethnicity, genetic endowment, the environment and the type of food available in local contexts. Were these problems of generalization of nutrition studies be substantial they would call for more sound research and more caution in universal rules about what is desirable to eat.

In addition, eating is not like taking pills. We eat for a number of reasons and the act of eating has a major role in our personal and social life. It is thus naïve to assume that evidence on what is good or bad, provided is really available, can easily translate into individual choices. How to motivate people to change nutrition behaviour requires a major effort in scientific fields that are more social than biomedical. Good science in psychology, sociology, anthropology and economics are needed to offer guidance about what can motivate people to eat less and better.

In sum, if we want to be serious about nutrition policy, better research and much more resources to do it are strongly needed. The analytical approach used to study individual nutrients and their mixes in diets is certainly useful. But as it is well shown in this original book, understanding the whole picture of eating and its implications from a broader scientific perspective are very warranted as well.

Prof. Giovanni Fattore, PhD
Department of Policy Analysis and Public Management, and CERGAS
Università Bocconi, Milano

The Author

Christopher Emsden has been a journalist for more than two decades in Italy, the U.S., Spain and Eastern Europe, most of them covering economic policies for the Wall Street Journal, the Economist Intelligence Unit and other publications. Raised in rural Colorado and now living in Rome with his wife and daughter, he trained as an anthropologist, doing fieldwork among so-called "pariah" castes in southern India, which catalyzed his interest in the way social hierarchies are blind to the long biological shadows they cast.

1 Ad Libitum

It is a miracle that one does not dissolve in one's bath like a lump of sugar.

Pablo Picasso

Somewhere, perhaps right now, a person is climbing 51 meters high in a tree to collect honey, a poignant example of how much we want sugar. That person would be a Pygmy in the Congo basin, and the tenacity of their purpose is underscored by the substantial mortality rate caused by falling from the jungle crown, not to mention the African bees' aggressive defense of their hives. Moreover, generations of genetic selection produced their short stature – an average adult is around 4 feet 7 inches – which is a huge asset when it comes to climbing. Evidence of a serious sweet tooth has been found in cave paintings, in the tombs of Egyptian pharaohs, in Sanskrit texts, on the walls of ancient Spanish cave paintings, and among contemporary peoples deep in the Amazon basin.

Most of us, of course, barely have to move a finger to eat something sweet, and so increasingly we don't, and in general end up consuming rather a lot of it. So today sugar, despite its formidable contribution to romance over the ages, is increasingly cast as a demonic villain that with industrial precision and speed is turning humans into stigmatized, diabetic, fat, and medically expensive people.

Official bodies are increasingly listening to its critics and suggesting that human consumption of sugar must be cut, drastically, or the world will face fiscal Armageddon in terms of public health care costs already destined to rise due to a host of other causes ranging from pollution to longer life spans.

A decade ago the World Health Organization (WHO) recommended that added sugars be capped at 10 percent of an individual's dietary energy intake. Now, with that target unachieved, it is recommending dropping it to 5 percent. And a prominent anti-obesity campaigner has suggested that it really must be slashed to 3 percent or dentists will ineluctably have to bankrupt us all. Such drastic appeals raise a host of questions, ranging from assessing the magnitude and trend of obesity to how to tackle it. Will regulation of a single food force improvement, or are there deeper causes beyond individual lifestyles to address?

Sugar has always been, tangentially, a big player in human history and social discourse. Its classic taste, sweetness, is shorthand for pleasure, the merits of which were debated long ago by the Greeks, with Plato decrying it as an illusion and Aristotle assuming it as part of human happiness and virtue. Today, sugar is seen as something that needs to be taken away from us, its pleasure an unaffordable luxury as the world's population is projected to grow to more than 9 billion in 2050, five times more than in 1900. Ironically, the quest for strategies to feed the world has heightened awareness that obesity, a form of malnourishment that can lead to illnesses such as Type 2 diabetes, is a global threat.

Fat, as in animal fat, was once deemed the cause, but dietary authorities have recently withdrawn that accusation, and now refined carbohydrates – especially the high-energy carbohydrate known as sugar – are in the dock as the cause.

Sugar's impact on the body has long been of note. Blackened teeth became a status symbol after sugar arrived as a luxury good in Elizabethan England, prompting aspiring penny-pinching social climbers to paint their own black for important dinner parties – a custom known in Japan as *ohaguro*. Far more than dental health was at stake when Tokyo banned it in 1870 as part of a systematic dismantling of feudal patterns, as *ohaguro* had long served as a signaling device, once for girls planning elite marriages of political convenience, and later a prerogative for aristocratic males. Later, anti-slavery activists staged campaigns against sugar, and after the Haitian Revolution in 1811 made obtaining cane more complicated for France, Napoleon ordered a vast expansion of sugar beets to produce it at home. That event, which was repeated across the temperate zone in countries such as the United States, Russia and Germany, was "a great service rendered by science to humanity, and furnishes an example which cannot but have the happiest results," wrote

Jean Anthelme Brillat-Savarin, the genial French gourmet whose *The Physiology of Taste: Or, Transcendental Gastronomy* was published in 1825.

His judgment is now in question. The internet is full of personal trainers and weight-loss gurus declaring that sugar is a killer, often citing studies based on astronomical consumption levels that are far above the norm, although certainly available. Magazine articles abound, usually with punning headline purporting to tell the "bitter truth about sugar" or reveal a number of "deadly truths."

Robert Lustig, a pediatric endocrinologist in San Francisco, has famously claimed sugar is in fact toxic, and more than 5.6 million people have clicked on his hour-and-a-half presentation on YouTube. Such stunning levels of interest show that people are increasingly convinced that something is rotten in the world, and the focus on food systems as the likely source is a classic symptom of social alarm and potential upheaval.

An admirably tireless crusader, Dr. Lustig hints that merely tweaking recommended daily allowances is not the major change in thinking that is needed in the face of the "obesity pandemic." His ideal recipe would be far more incisive – the removal of sugar from the list of food additives such as garlic, basil and vitamin A that are "generally regarded as safe."

Referring to the American Declaration of Independence in his new book, *Fat Chance: The Hidden Truth About Sugar, Obesity and Disease,* he writes: "We are entitled to life, liberty and the pursuit of happiness. It doesn't say a damned fucking thing about the pursuit of pleasure."

That constitutional concept of happiness tracks back to John Locke, who in his seventeenth-century "Essay Concerning Human Understanding" saw "the necessity of pursuing happiness [as] the foundation of liberty," and then sagely slipped in a clause distinguishing "imaginary" and "true" happiness to build a notion in which the human skill of abstinence is deployed as the handrail on the stairway to heaven.

Bluntly put, happiness and freedom are universal rights, but only a select few are able to define what they are in practice. That immediately raises the question of which caste of experts has the best purchase on "true happiness" and there are no shortage of candidates in the running. Regarding sugar, for instance, there are a panoply of factions among nutritional scientists, a group not known for consensus and which does not always see eye to eye with the medical community, itself split between researchers and clinicians; and then there are farmers, refiners, commercial users and, finally, the people who eat it, with their myriad interests and social obligations.

Efforts to translate a "true" definition of happiness and liberty to the world of actual goods highlights how much is at stake. Restrictions on access to goods could, for example, amount to removing the aforementioned handrail on the stairway in favor of a conveyor belt and then declaring the areas next to it off limits to pedestrians. They represent a rather authoritarian view wherein the individual is assumed to be unable to move beyond what Locke would call the "animal state," enslaved to passions, and unable to distinguish properly between imaginary and true pleasures.

Removing sugar from the list of legal foods will also relieve many parents of the task of telling their children that they can't have the chocolate egg in the supermarket, because the eggs will be removed. That no doubt may offer some immediate relief to harried parents, but it also strips away the learning process postulated as the only real way to distinguish true from false happiness.

Indeed, it is striking how many sugar demonizers today seek a drastic curtailment of sugar in the food system rather than more incisive labeling requirements. That belies a loss of faith in education as a tool for public health. It may seem like it is not effective, but perhaps it is not being pursued or distributed effectively. At any rate, spurning the role of education may create some unexpected reactions.

Here an interesting example helps underscore the point.

Insofar as children are assumed not to be responsible for the material context of their lives, restraints on their freedom of action may make sense, and various initiatives have used this logic to ban sugar-heavy foods and drinks from schools. This is generally championed as smart – "a common sense cure to obesity" in the words of the WHO.

But there is scant evidence that such measures lead to weight loss or even reduced sugar consumption of the youths involved, who often simply pick up a soda or two on their way home from school. But some more intriguing forms of resistance suggest the cure may leave the designated patients worse off than the presumed risk they face.

In the wake of reports that a third of British youth were overweight or obese, Parliament passed a rule restricting the sale on public school sites of cookies, chips, sweetened drinks, chocolate, and confectionery items. What ensued is a proliferating black market that exacerbated existing social tensions and served as an induction mechanism for youths to learn the arts of illicit trade, as well as channeling revenue to supermarkets. Kids basically smuggled doughnuts, candy, energy drinks, and biscuits in and sold them to colleagues at a profit on campus, often after having arranged the sale via their smartphones – according to Adam Fletcher, a professor at Cardiff University, who led the study based on data and interviews from students aged 12 and up at six secondary schools spanning the socioeconomic spectrum of the more affluent parts of the country.

The typical markup was generally seen as "reasonable" both by sellers and buyers, said Fletcher, who for a decade worked at the London School of Hygiene & Tropical Medicine (LSHTM), one of the world's foremost research institutions for public health issues.

He also noted that kids appeared quite deliberative about their collective reaction to the new law, citing one 15-year-old girl as saying: "We've got some underground business selling junk food. It is just the school can't force you to do anything." In a rich jibe to those who made the rule, she added: "You need to be more educated with it."

In the end, a presumably well-meaning and apparently common-sense policy appears to have led to a situation where access to the unhealthy food in question has increased, where kids learn to break the rules – and so do the teaching staff, who recognized the widespread practice and in some cases actively participated – and where the evident potential analogy to illegal drug trading was increasingly recognized as teenagers neared the point of leaving school. On top of that, many students used their profits to eat fast food in the afternoon!

Overweight in particular has a long history of failed solutions. As it happens, obesity was quite an issue around the turn of the twentieth century, a time of major social change when "thinness had become a way in which young privileged women could distance themselves from their working-class counterparts."[1]

Data are scant but popular media took up the theme, and there were of course fads like the notion that drinking water was fattening – so at times were potatoes and bananas – or that chewing a lot and eating only one kind of food at a meal would make you thin. Exercise was timidly mentioned from time to time. Gradually, sociological forces focused the message mainly on women.

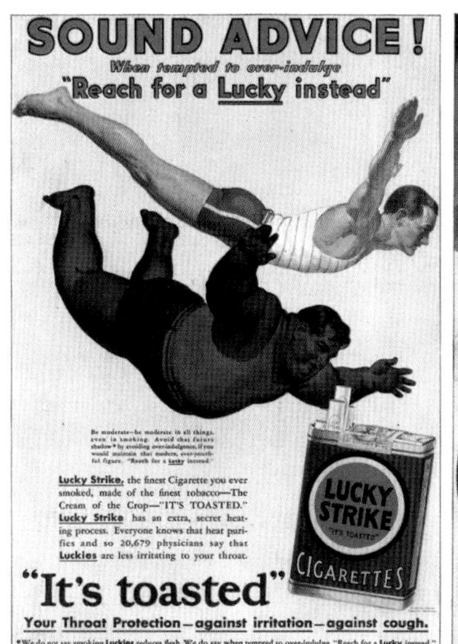

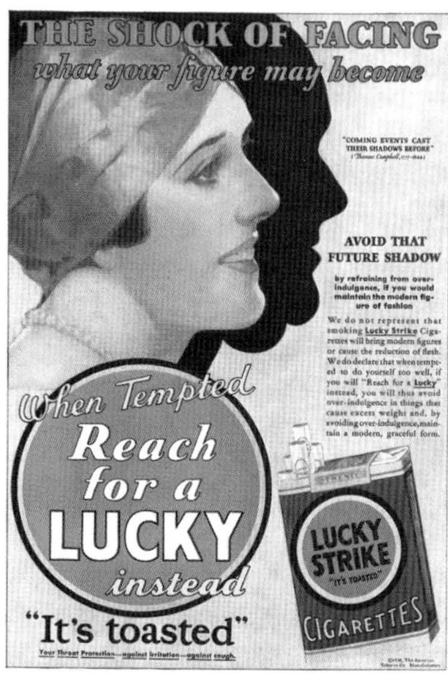

Smoking cigarettes was pitched as a way to win the battle of the bulge in these advertisements from the 1920s and 1930s

Source: From the collection of Stanford University (tobacco.stanford.edu)

Eventually sugar entered the fray as a choice target. "Avoid temptation" became a slogan often seen on billboards and magazine advertisements. Their sponsors were tobacco companies.

Quick fixes

While tobacco brought a host of new health problems and challenged social mores, nicotine is a proven appetite suppressant and those who switched made a trade-off that may have produced benefits uncaptured by the medical tally. Keeping slim almost certainly enhanced a young woman's position in the matrimonial arena, itself being vastly revolutionized by urbanization. *Ohaguro* redux!

Trade-offs pose challenging personal and policy questions, as often experts operate with benchmarks that assume consumers face a more frictionless array of choices than we individuals actually feel we have. In the early twentieth century, Georges d'Avenel, a French viscount, gave popular lectures in Paris and New York on what he called the "leveling out" of enjoyment between classes, telling his peers that tolerating equal access to small luxuries was preferable to the equalization of incomes and deploring as a contradiction the snobbish attitude of hailing the genius of human industry while deploring its consumerist results.

Restricting sweet-and-salty "comfort foods," on the grounds of their poor nutritional quality, without tackling the systemic social or personal stress their prevalence reflects may end up stripping away people's right to the pursuit of plausible happiness rather than just pleasure.

Informed choices, of course, are better than the other kind. Yet achieving credibility as a purveyor of official information may be harder at times of rapid social change. Calling for drastic cuts to sugar consumption may ultimately only amount to an exercise in visibility which stokes latent distrust in all claims and encourages sectarian commitments rather than community health.

Indeed, in the postwar era, as health authorities waged battle against smoking – which in North America interestingly peaked well before the anti-cigarette push reached a regulatory crescendo – sugar rebounded by claiming no other food offers satiety with so few calories. "Are you getting enough sugar to keep your weight down?" asked one advertisement, acknowledging that the proposal "sounds strange."

Today such a claim seems like the height of sophistry – technically correct, perhaps, but somehow missing the point – and it is useful to keep that rhetorical genre in mind while mulling the war over sugar. Today, a slew of sophisticated lobbies fight it out, with pharmaceutical and food companies disagreeing on sugar's health effects, while internecine battles proliferate between companies that use sugar, companies that offer alternative sweeteners and companies that refine sugar, not to mention producers of sugar cane or maize whose byproducts can be churned into high-fructose corn syrup, another form of $C_{12}H_{22}O_{11}$, sucrose's chemical signature.

A category implodes

Given the popular demonization of sugar it is interesting to note that it still has plenty of brand value, and not just as a popular if somewhat quaint term of endearment.

The Western Sugar Cooperative, representing around 1,000 US sugar beet farmers, joined with similar firms in 2011 to sue the Corn Refiners Association (CRA) for false advertising with its marketing of high-fructose corn syrup (HFCS) as "corn sugar." In essence, they wanted the word for themselves, even though their own product was itself developed as a substitute for sugar cane.

CRA President Audrae Erickson dismissed the allegations, saying: "Sugar is sugar. High fructose corn syrup and sugar are nutritionally and metabolically equivalent." In 2012, her organization then countersued The Sugar Association, accusing it of deceiving consumers into believing that processed sugar is safer and more healthful than HFCS and adding that "vilifying one kind of added sugar will not reduce Americans' waistlines."

While it is fashionable to blame all sorts of woes on some generic lobby – Big Food, Big Pharma, Wall Street – in this case we are witness to an exquisitely internecine battle inside one of these putative monoliths. It could be depicted as an implosion – even a form of metabolic syndrome – happening inside the world of sugar itself, one featuring role reversals and revealing dynamic changes not only in understanding but also potentially in the way things function. Similar shifts are taking place in the scientific worlds of genetics and microbiology that are certain to lead to new thoughts about medicine and nutrition.

Half a million pages of evidence have been submitted to the US District Court in Los Angeles, and high-profile trial lawyers have been engaged. The docket shows the plaintiffs also linked the syrup to the "obesity epidemic,"[2] a high-risk strategy that may make the eventual sentence a landmark ruling.

It has not been an easy time for the CRA, as not only did the federal court dismiss its attempted countersuit, but the Food and Drug Administration (FDA) decided in 2012 to deny its petition to call HFCS "corn sugar." The FDA explained its decision by noting that, according to the dictionary and under its regulatory approach, sugars are solids and syrups are liquids.[3]

Referring to the sugar industry as a cartel now seems rather preposterous. As the above conflict points out, the gloves are off between two clans in the sweetener business, which itself doesn't always have placid relations with branded food companies, the opaque world of flavor synthesizers and of course the world of actual stores, where changes are driving big upstream mutations in the business fabric such as H.J. Heinz Co. taking over and merging with Kraft Foods Group Inc. in a bid to bulk up and push back against retail superpowers. There has also been lasting tension between American sugar producers and food manufacturers after a government report noted that for each agricultural job saved by domestic price supports, nearly three jobs in the confectionery sector were lost in just five years.[4]

Moreover, big changes are looming as the European Union (EU) prepares to dismantle its sugar market protections, putting pressure on the US to follow suit. Commodities experts presume Brazil, far and away the biggest sugar producer, will be the big winner. But there will be another effect that might matter to those pitching healthish ideas like sin taxes on sodas or promoting no-calorie sweeteners. European food companies can expect sugar prices to drop by a quarter, and US firms by even more.

Whatever form and price sugar ends up having, it has glucose, which happens to be the brain's sole source of energy. Successful human craving for sugar was an evolutionary asset and instrumental in developing the bigger brains that led our species to stand up and, eventually, dominate the planet. Many scientists endorse the notion that we live in the Anthropocene geological era, although there is robust debate about exactly when we started calling the shots. The implication is that we now have no choice but to redraw traditional distinctions between nature and nurture, between genetic and environmental causes, or between purely nutritional and social causes. It may even be that life in the Anthropocene, or at least since the birth of agriculture around 10,000 years ago, requires smaller brains – meaning that, just as the Pygmies' short stature is adaptive to agile tree climbing for honey, we would be better off with fewer neurons from now on. The ultimate reason for the call to deprogram our sugar craving and intake may be to help dumb ourselves down! Perhaps the relentless forces of urbanization will force sugar cane, which today produces more calories per acre than any other crop in the world, to retreat back to its genetic homeland on the island of Papua New Guinea, considered its genetic homeland and widely grown there as a garden crop.

A world in which a few forest holdouts enjoy sugar rushes would be ripe for satirical treatment along the lines of the 1995 film *Waterworld* with its cigarette-smoking pirates upsetting future humans' efforts to restore a bit of precious soil. But perhaps some might find it more fun to make a sequel to *The Matrix* and concentrate on the billions of sugar-free urban foodies hewing to stringent health and nutrition regulations, cutting back their screen time, engaging in ample outdoor exercise and shipping in the ingredients of the fashionable Paleolithic diet – meat, nuts, and fresh fruit, but no processed food like cheese or wine or pasta – as remote sensors monitor the biodiversity in their gut.

A diet without cheap carbohydrates might however be more of a solution for a privileged elite than for all of us, which again raises the question of true happiness. After all, the *Scientific Report* of the US government's 2015 Dietary Guidelines Advisory Committee, in reviewing the state of research on added sugars and body weight, noted that a correlation appeared typical of "free-living people consuming ad libitum." That's the way nutrition scientists refer to prosperous liberal societies that face no constraints on food intake. I must confess here that my initial impression of the phrase was that it represented a highly consensual view of a desirable state, which is what it is meant to be. However, it turns out that a lot of people have misgivings.

Ad libitum, Latin for at one's pleasure or liberty, is generally used to mean ad lib or improvisation in theatrical contexts. The term is also the canonical description of how rats used in laboratory experiments are fed.

It's important to note that such rats in no way experience the first part of the dietary guidelines' boilerplate. They live in fairly crowded cages after all, and live sedentary lives with "virtually no environmental stimulation," as noted in an important research paper published by the *Proceedings of the National Academy of Sciences*.[5] These rats – the ones used as benchmarks, not their brethren who are subjected to tests – are already overweight and glucose intolerant. Simply cutting their access to chow pellets vastly increases their longevity and reduces their disease incidence.

Hopefully people, who have many environmental exposures both positive and negative in terms of health, are different, and that is largely due to the "free living" part of the *ad libitum* phrase. As for cutting back on food in general, Luigi Cornaro wrote a whole book some 500 years ago on how his spartan diet along with caraffes of wine helped him live past his hundredth birthday.

Sugar as a nearly primordial form of glucose is one of the original superfoods, inevitably triggering strong opinions because at the end of the day food is one thing we all need and share. As Brillat-Savarin noted, every social force gathers around the table, including "love, friendship, business, speculation, power, importunity, patronage, ambition, intrigue." This book's theme is that sugar is but a pawn on a chessboard where multiple forces are battling over how to cope with broader evolutionary, environmental, social, economic, medical, scientific, and technological changes emerging in today's world – a world full of noble intentions, dirty tricks and surprising new discoveries.

A warning on style

This book is written by a journalist and anthropologist, not a nutritionist or professor of public health.

It was conceived of as a way of exploring why we are so uneasy about our modern food system, and while it always aspired to be an essay rather than a report, its eventual form represents a surprise compared to assumptions made at the outset, which were mainly that sugar, so white and refined, had a dark story stretching from slavery and perhaps all the way to ongoing toxic abuse. Slavery did exist, the author is baffled that anyone lets infants drink soda, and agrees that eating more leafy vegetables and fewer hyper-processed foods would be a fine individual choice. But there is a veritable tsunami of evidence that its role in obesity is a bit-part in a much more complex and at times troubling drama.

It was surprising to realize that, even though the WHO reviewed 17,000 scientific papers – albeit ultimately discarding 99.6 percent of them – before arriving at its suggestion to further curtail recommended intakes, the idea that sugar is more than a high-energy ultra-refined carbohydrate still remains conjecture.[6]

What is clear, by contrast, is that metabolic disorders disproportionately emerge most where people face disruptive and unsought social and cultural changes that themselves embody timeworn human flaws and increasingly also reflect ecological stresses due to what Pope Francis called "rapidification." That word aptly describes not only aspects of the way modern food is consumed, but the evolutionary setting in which pollinating insects and many wild animals live today, and too often also the way we treat each other.

The title of this book, *Sweetness and Light,* does not refer to sugar but to the method of inquiry. It aspires to refer to an attitudinal style endorsed by Matthew Arnold, the iconic High Victorian who defined culture as "a study of perfection" and warned that many a critic is really "but a man with a system, an advocate." In his central work, *Culture and Anarchy,* he said his approach would be one of "getting to know, on all the matters which most concern us, the best which has been thought and said in the world, and through this knowledge, turning a stream of fresh and free thought upon our stock notions and habits." The phrase continues: "which we now follow staunchly but mechanically, vainly imagining that there is a virtue in following them staunchly which makes up for the mischief of following them mechanically." Arnold has fallen out of fashion, but it is worth noting that in the late nineteenth century – a time he described in a poem as one of "wandering between two worlds, one dead, the other powerless to be born" – he was trying to pacify the ideological tumult of his time by establishing distinct roles for science and religion, one in which the former was identified as a humanistic art and the latter an ethic of "duty, self-control and hard work."

That, anyway, is the aspiration.

Due disclosure: "sweetness and light" was first used in English by Jonathan Swift, in *The Battle of the Books,* a spoofy 1704 mock dialogue about the respective merits of the ancient and modern learning in which, as it happens, the key scene consists of a spider arguing with a bee about metabolic matters. The spider claims to be a creative type, spinning fabulous webs from internal fibers, while the bee claims to be a selfless altruist and regards the filaments really as consisting of bits of dirt along with flies digested after being infected by poison.

Swift is of course best known for his later essay, "A Modest Proposal," which suggested that poor Irish people – whose conditions the native Dubliner described in great detail – might fare better if they sold their children to the elite as food.

That was irony, to be sure, and squarely aimed at the vogue for simple solutions.

Purgatory 2

Sanity is not statistical.
George Orwell

"We need grains, salt and sugar." That was the appeal by Ram Sharan Mahat, Nepal's finance minister, after his country was rocked by an earthquake measuring 7.9 on the Richter scale that killed thousands of people and left many more short of food in 2015. All the items on his wish list would be frowned upon by nutrition police, but his request underscored how they remain fundamental staples in the human food supply.

Sugar, for example, plays a large role in preservation and palatability, making it a core ingredient in processed foods, a category that ranges from wine and olive oil to Pringles Baked Wheat Stix Crispy Cracker Pizza Sticks. Its ubiquity – multiplied by the fact that human digestion quickly breaks all sorts of food into basic sugars – may be the main reason it is being targeted as a possible cause of contemporary ailments.

That sugar is under attack can be illustrated by an internet search. Typing in "sugar" and "health" brings up about 340 million results in 0.38 seconds on Google's search engine, more than tobacco and pollution combined and two times more than "poverty and health" elicits.

The tone of the entry headings is suggestive. A search keyed to tobacco and health calls up a slew of fact sheets – technical documents with few adjectives. Google pollution and health and again mostly governmental sites linking the two in calm tones pop up. For sugar and health, meanwhile, the headlines use attention-grabbing and suggestive phrases like "sweet poison," "harmful effects," "ruin," "death" and the inevitable "ten things you don't know."

Search optimization is an advanced art, but for the record, the first sentence of the first entry reads: "Added sugar is the single worst ingredient in the modern diet" and says it contributes "to all sorts of diseases." The article appears on a website named Authority Nutrition with a dot com domain that prominently features four meal plans "that can save your life."[1]

The density of a Google search correlates to the liveliness of a debate, and so it is in this case. Fat is yesterday's demon, and gluten is only a minor devil in today's nutritionism. And that's because, as things stand, science is not settled when it comes to sugar. No causal link between sugar and diabetes mellitus has been discovered, nor to any other non-communicable diseases.

What is known is that eating more than you use – regardless of the food – will usually lead to weight gain, and on that front it can be added that sugar is a very efficient source of energy. It would be hard to get fat on kale because it would be hard to pack enough away into digestibly usable calories.

Obesity, a broader term referring to a condition that may or may not be a disease,[2] can result from excess consumption of various food items including sugar. No standard definition of obesity exists, and while the Body Mass Index (BMI) is ubiquitous in public health journals, professionals concur that it is at best an heuristic device. According to the WHO, worldwide obesity, measured in BMI terms, has more than doubled since 1980 and now affects more than 600 million adults. Add in overweight and 39 percent of the global population has a BMI above 25, deemed a major risk factor for diabetes, heart disease, and stroke, as well as various cancers and other ailments. The WHO also estimates that 347 million people, or 9 percent of the world's adult population, have diabetes – half of them unaware of the fact – and that the number of diabetes deaths will double between 2005 and 2030, by which time it will be the world's seventh leading cause of death. Reducing the prevalence of diabetes is achievable, it says, through lower body weights, physical exercise, and a diet comprising more fruit and vegetables and less sugar and saturated fats.

While scores of scientific and medical investigations have pointed to correlations between excess sugar consumption and Type 2 diabetes, they invariably acknowledge a host of contingent factors that might be primary causes. The increase in obesity and diabetes is a global phenomenon and appears to correlate tightly with broader industrial and especially urbanization patterns which can introduce a host of economic, local, lifestyle, and psychological changes as well as impact on evolutionary processes directly.

Obesity is a classic case of a "wicked problem," meaning it is difficult to define, is socially complex, and likely has multiple and interdependent causes, making it highly resistant to any clear solution. Wicked problems invariably open up a Pandora's box – they are, in a way, themselves symptoms of other problems, some of which have offered great benefits over time. As they entail thickly-woven and consequential tradeoffs, solutions are tricky and can lead to unexpected surprises.

Consider the automobile, which revolutionized lifestyles, comfort and logistics, and also contributed to lower levels of physical activity, all of which are implicated in weight gain. Cars and trucks enabled a revolution in food systems ranging from farming to shopping. Traffic accidents and driving stress ensued, as did predatory car loans, gas station minimarkets and of course pollution – which has a particularly intense relation to obesity. It turns out that maternal exposure to air pollution – especially in poor urban neighborhoods such as the Bronx – makes childhood obesity twice as likely already by the age of 5. Separate research, based on a long-term cohort in southern California and looking at developments from the age of 5 to 11, also found that air pollution predisposes kids themselves towards obesity, a finding matched by experiments with laboratory rats. The same team, led by Michael Jerrett, a professor at the University of California in Berkeley, then found the same pattern applied to children from 10 to high-school graduation at 18.[3]

Air pollution is apparently even more problematic for obesity trends, as yet newer research has just shown that people who are already obese in fact breathe in up to 50 percent more air than those who are not – and it's almost 25 percent for obese children – setting off a self-perpetuating doomsday loop. Very heavy adults often breathe in half as much air every day as Tour de France cyclists do during their peak performance according to Pierre Brochu, a professor of public health at the University of Montreal and lead author of that study.

While all scientists love to point out that more research is necessary, much has been done. For example, the set of chemicals known as polycyclic aromatic hydrocarbons – released into the air via car exhaust but also via forest fires and using the grill to cook food – can even at very low doses block the process of lipolysis in mice, meaning that fats are not broken down but rather stored in excess adipose tissue. There are also 800 known endocrine disruptors – chemicals used in agriculture and industry that can crawl into adipocyte cells and disrupt metabolism, and many have not been tested, according to a 2015 report on planetary health by the Rockefeller Foundation and *The Lancet* medical journal.

In short, one of the very plausible stories behind the obesity pandemic is that it is driven by Anthropocene factors such as use of motor vehicles and operates by physiological disruptions that do not depend on the food chain at all.

Moreover, the effect of air pollution is vastly greater on the poor than the wealthy, which correlates all too well with obesity itself. Two recent studies have conducted fine-grained geographic analysis of the unequal and iniquitous way that air pollution is distributed in the USA. Given that those analyses are keyed to the relative intensity of local unequal exposures rather than absolute clinical levels, it is striking how they broadly resemble the national map of obesity itself.[4]

The foregoing consideration[5] suggests there are strong social factors in the epidemiology of disease, rendering quite suggestive the term "social metabolism" coined by Karl Marx long ago to refer to what he saw as a rupture in the interaction between humanity and the rest of nature that he noted at a time – we are in the mid-1800s – of sharply accelerating urbanization across Europe. Marx typically focused on how capitalism impacted modes of production and, interestingly enough, one of the big changes happening in European agriculture at the time was major innovation – through agricultural chemistry and also through colonialism – in the use of soil fertilizers.

The word "metabolism" moved fairly quickly from referring just to human digestive processes to something larger, spurred by Justus von Liebig's groundbreaking work on organic chemistry, wherein he noted that urbanization entailed, among other things, the one-way transfer of nitrogen, phosphorous, and potassium – all crucial soil elements for farming – to the cities where people ate the foods the farms produced but did not return the soil nutrients. That metabolic syndromes reflect a set of factors extending well beyond diet is also suggested by evidence that domesticated animals show signs resembling diabetes, perhaps the price of protection from predators. That something of the same nature may be true for the modern human species as well is an updated variant of why some people refer to cardiovascular ailments as diseases of affluence or civilization.

Playing the numbers

Civilization, of course, changes. Sugar is an example, as it became widely available to Europeans during the course of the nineteenth century, not least thanks to brutal plantation regimes in many tropical countries. Yet while sugar consumption had risen to a striking level in western societies already by 1900, other changes were yet to come.

Consider the fate of eating at home, once a defining social fact of human life but now often skipped due to increasingly irregular work schedules. For most Americans, the three-meals-a-day paradigm has been supplanted by the five-snacking-sessions mode, and while that now involves a deluge of energy-dense "junk food" and in some cases even expensive high-nutrient vegetable juices, it is just an example of contemporary food systems profitably catering to a trend whose wicked roots must surely lie elsewhere.[6]

As today's demonization of sugar is linked essentially to growing obesity, it is imperative to assess whether this is a real or somewhat imaginary crisis, and whether it is really a symptom of a much broader panic over nutrition and food in general. And while we all share practical interest in possible solutions to a problem that allegedly is already costing the world almost $3 trillion a year – almost as much as armed violence, war, and terrorism according to an "initial economic analysis" recently put forth by the McKinsey consultancy firm[7] – we must consider how history shows that human triumphs over endemic diseases have tended to come when new discoveries upend previous understandings.

So what is the reason for the panic over obesity, which started its ascent from a sleepy subject to a media fixture in the late 1980s?

As it turns out, the dramatic story of surging weight problems as told by the numbers – especially when described as percentages compared to earlier eras – relies on a benchmark index that has not been stable. The BMI is a measure of one's weight in kilograms divided by the square of one's height in meters. The key BMI metric above which one is classified as overweight is now 25, but until recently it was 27.1, according to the US government's agriculture and health departments. That numerical switch pushed 37 million Americans into the overweight category before they even had time to shirk physical activity or eat another donut!

A similar story applies to setting 30 as the BMI threshold beyond which one is obese, a classification whose ranks have tripled among

US men since 1960. Given that clinical practitioners note that patients often become less engaged in weight-loss regimes when told they are obese, this is a handle-with-care issue, especially as obviously the great majority of people in the stigmatized category likely have a BMI in the low 30s. Fewer than one in five "obese" Americans has a BMI above 40, when health complications intensify greatly.

The way numbers are used in public health debates can be bewildering. For example, a 30 percent gap emerges in estimated prevalence depending on which of the two main indicators is used today, fasting plasma glucose score or HbA1c, a measure of glycated hemoglobin. That comes on top of the lowering of that and other metabolic indicators which had already greatly increased the number of putative diabetic cases. By one count, reclassification of cutoffs implied that 75 percent of Americans were diseased and should be taking medicines, and that was back in 1999![8]

Numbers jump around in media reports about obesity as well, obscuring what appears likely, which is that obesity in the U.S. appears to have broadly stabilized since 2000 except for the relatively small class of so-called morbidly obese.

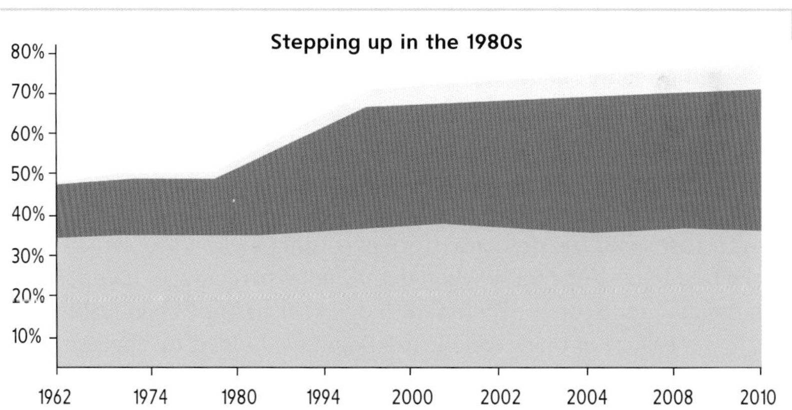

The American body profile – the color lines in the chart show BMI above 25, 30 and 40 respectively – changed sharply from 1980 through 1997. Possible reasons range from dietary changes, new classification methods, or perhaps that people born in the Depression passed the age of 50

Source: National Institute of Diabetes and Digestive and Kidney Diseases

Using the new BMI cutoffs, some 46 percent of American adults were overweight or obese already in 1962, a figure which rose to almost 70 percent by 2000 and has since leveled off, according to this chart from the National Institute of Diabetes and Digestive and Kidney Diseases. The category of extreme obesity rose fivefold, from one percent to five percent, while the obesity category grew to 31 percent from 13 percent.

The second trend, offering hope that the remarkable run-up in the 1980s and 1990s is over, affects the vast majority of US citizens and must surely be welcomed – especially the 2014 report from federal health authorities that the rate of obesity among children aged two to five has dropped a giant 43 percent in the past decade.[9] Meanwhile, the *International Journal of Obesity Research*, published by World Obesity, the new name for an advocacy group formed in the 1970s that has had remarkable influence in drafting WHO guidelines, reported that the prevalence of a BMI above 40 has risen a whopping 70 percent since 2000, with even faster growth for those with BMIs above 50.

Perusing the statistical annex to the latter paper, however, one notes that only around 0.5 percent of Americans have a BMI above 50. Rightly noting the data are based on self-reported height and weight and that people may have a tendency to massage the figures a bit, the authors opted to make an adjustment that in fact increased by more than 50 percent the incidence of BMI above 40, thus generating most of the growth they report.

One of the authors has since published an analysis positing that obesity rates have risen for all American social groups in step with increased leisure time, increased exercise habits, and increased availability of fresh fruit and vegetables. He suggests targeted taxes levied on some foods could nudge behaviors towards healthier diets and that clinicians should act as opinion-leaders to bolster political support for such interventions.[10]

There are a few key takeaways from the contrasting emphases of the above two analyses: first, almost half of Americans were classified as heavier than they should be more than 50 years ago; second, the first Wal-Mart store had yet to open then; third, there was a significant jump in obesity in the 1980s and 1990s, uncannily coinciding with a time when average hourly labor wages began to decline in real terms and unemployment benefits tightened; fourth, extreme obesity is a condition that is unlikely to be caused by candy alone and which, while serious, is currently about as high as the number of Americans who want to undergo an operation to change their gender,[11] thus possibly not warranting use of the term "pandemic"; and fifth, one must keep an eye out for the rhetoric of numbers, as the "doubling in a decade" and "0.5 percent" are likely to make deliberately differing contributions to public awareness and debate.

The BMI – a simple calculation of one's weight divided by one's height squared – was developed as an intellectual exercise in the 1830s by Adolphe Quetelet, a Belgian mathematician interested in predictive models of astronomical phenomena, on the basis of information about French and Scottish men drafted into the military. It was then developed by the insurance industry, which by definition is interested in large-scale statistical correlations rather than specific health dynamics. Although rarely discussed in the media, it turns out that lower-than-average BMIs have a slightly higher mortality rate – the critical indicator par excellence! – than higher ones and that the danger mark is when BMIs go above 35 - which translates to a weight of about 240 pounds for the average American man, who is 5 feet 9 inches tall.

As it happens, most professional National Football League players are obese by this metric, and half of them extremely so, rates far above the population who consume beer and corn chips while watching them on television.[12]

On the other end of the spectrum, pastoralist herder communities along with hunter and gatherer groups are those who tend to have the lowest BMIs, coming in at around 21 on average, with considerable variation. It should be noted that traditional lifestyles with low BMIs by no means have shared dietary characteristics, and some in arctic regions take in an exceptionally high share of fats. For the record, the Hazda people in Tanzania rank honey as their preferred food, above meat or berries, or the low-calorie tubers they grudgingly eat when nothing else is available.[13]

Of course, the average life expectancy of hunters and gatherers is well short of that achieved in industrialized nations. That said, the difference may be much less if compared to western societies a few centuries ago. Longevity of the Hazda and similar peoples appears to be roughly the same as in eighteenth-century Sweden, and once early childhood mortality is excluded, the gap between contemporary America is far narrower than the overall figure suggests.[14]

The same applies – albeit in reverse – to captive chimpanzees, who benefit from medical attention, secure food supplies, and protection from predation and consequently have much higher survival rates while young than their brethren in the wild. Curiously, that fades and reverses as they age, again possibly pointing to some adverse health effect of domestication. Purely dietary facts show that *Homo sapiens* is remarkably diverse, able to live in vastly differing natural environments and adjust their macronutrient profiles accordingly, sometimes living primarily on animal products – seal comprised 80 percent of the traditional diet of some northern Inuit peoples – other times relying massively on carbohydrates, as in swathes of Asia devoted to rice. Indeed, in terms of dietary shares of energy coming from protein, fat, and carbohydrates respectively, the modern American diet – chosen here because of the heightened public alarm over obesity – is smack in the middle of a comparative panorama including primates, nomadic groups, pastoralists, and traditional agriculturalists. And in terms of daily energy intake – the famous calorie tally – Americans are also in the middle range and well below the typical intakes of coal miners and farmers of the not-so-distant western past.

So what's the fuss? Is the world heading to a health calamity? Might the noise be driven by fiscal fears related to the eventual health care costs of a world where people have longer life spans? Is it all a ploy to introduce new and profitable solutions just in time to allay the crisis, more or less using scary evocations of "risk factors" to drum up pharmaceutical prescriptions as many feel has been done with cholesterol-lowering statins? Might the epidemiology here stray far from the medical body and into social tactics?

The real epidemic, according to Paul Campos, a law professor at the University of Colorado, is in the explosion of claims that obesity is a serious public health problem. He calculated a hundredfold increase in the number of US news articles devoted to the word "obesity" from 1980 to 2004 and noted that many of them are triggered by reports coming from interested parties, often in the pharmaceutical or weight-loss industries. For Campos, we are witnessing a "moral panic," which "are typical during times of rapid social change and involve an exaggeration or fabrication of risks, the use of disaster analogies, and the projection of societal anxieties onto a stigmatized group."

His is a salutary contribution to the debate. Ironically, given he was questioning the actual existence of a health crisis – he suggested that weight gains among American adults really amounted to the equivalent of an extra Big Mac every two months that could be offset by a few minutes of walking very day and suggested obesity was a tool to berate minorities for not going to gyms or eating enough fresh produce – his fusillade may have ultimately helped prod a shift towards a new paradigm in which obesity remains what it in fact is, a serious problem, but one best seen as the outcome of systemic forces rather than the result of personal choices or any single cause.[15]

The warning that we are witnessing a "moral crisis" ought to be taken seriously. Many fields are now blamed for an array of woes based on deeply structural flaws. Finance, the alleged culprit of the global crisis that led to job destruction and bank bailouts with no known price tag, is a prime example. And even if we ignore reports that workers in the financial sector are more prone to lie and leave ethical questions out of the picture, there is no doubt that experts agree that a lucrative industry heavily populated by the best and brightest was out of whack due to eminently avoidable technical errors in design.

Apprehension about the effects of climate change are rife, spurring acrimonious accusations of lethal misbehavior. Often well-meaning champions of sustainable solutions clash due to differences in the scale of the solutions being sought, allowing advocates of perfection to discredit those pursuing mere improvement.

Take biofuels. The Global Renewable Fuels Alliance, a lobby comprising industry players, claims they are a precious and economical tool to reduce greenhouse gas emissions caused by crude oil. The World Resources Institute, a global non-profit think-tank devoted to environmental issues and a funding favorite of several European governments, released a 2015 report arguing that the cost of channeling food crops to fuel outweighed the benefits when the potential value of land was factored in and that their ultimate carbon benefits were overstated. So everyone acts out their assigned role, which can make it harder for a more nuanced case to be heard. In the end, a battle between big private interests and the global constituency affected by climate change may end up delegitimizing plans to make energy available where it is currently scarce.[16]

Attributing conflicting thoughts to lobbies is too reductive; what we do see, though, is a general lack of intellectual confidence in the institutions trusted with authority, leading to an increased skepticism about public solutions and a greater interest in the do-it-yourself kind.

Returning to the "moral crisis" surrounding obesity, it is a concern – researchers found that, in 2014, the majority of people who read a news story about obesity as a "public health crisis" had no reaction in terms of their perception of health risks but significantly increased their prejudice against fat people.[17]

Given the waves of scientific investigations suggesting that obesity is caused by systemic factors – excess sugar intake, for some, imbalances in our gut bacteria, for others, not to mention pollution and other factors touched on above – it's quite remarkable that we revert to such a simplified view.

If intensified public discourse on obesity leads to negative reactions – overweight people also tend to lose interest when they are told they are obese – then we are in the presence of a seemingly paradoxical mechanism whereby declaring an "epidemic" actually worsens the clinical environment and potentially undermines efforts to reach a welfare-enhancing settlement.

With such a backdrop, providing official guidance is a delicate balancing act, insofar as the aim is to achieve meaningful progress towards a given goal. If the goal is better health and nutrition, that will require sweeping changes – more school sports programs for all and higher income for many in exchange for less work to promote eating together as families, to list a few easy-to-see examples – that will not come easily nor cheaply.

Wicked problems, as noted above, are battles over both definitional facts and behavioral solutions. Are we sure of the scale of the obesity problem, and sure it won't self-correct on its own? Are we sure that carbohydrates, above all sugars, are the core drivers of weight gain, even where calorie intakes are middling and new discoveries are being made suggesting obesity is the result of a microbe deficit in our intestines? Are we sure it's food, and not deleterious social patterns linked to power and stress, that is the source of our panic, and illnesses?

Dante Alighieri, after having explored hell, begins the second tome of his *Divine Comedy* by urging himself to raise the sail of his own genius to tell the tale of Purgatory, where the human spirit "purges itself" and becomes worthy of an eventual ascent to heaven. Purgatory, a midway point between heaven and hell cannily invented in the Middle Ages, sets the right mood for an evidence-based approach to the future of our food and nutrition. Many feel our global food system has lost its way in a brambly thicket, but there is no scientific shortcut to heaven.

"The Birth of Purgatory," according to French historian Jacques Le Goff's subtle thesis, came about in the twelfth century as itself an innovative institution mediating the emergence of European social classes beyond the all-powerful aristocratic and ecclesiastical castes and the subaltern peasantry. Much as the concept of risk has emerged in public health discourse today as a constant negative designed to catalyze anxiety and compliance, Purgatory emerged as a wiggly way to accommodate more social diversity. It was where you went if, say, you tinkered with sin but were generally a good person. By essentially allowing for a few errors, it doubtless encouraged a bit of experimental science and progress. It was, as we'd say today, an inclusive multi-stakeholder-driven solution to a wicked problem at a time of social change. And it was cannily designed not merely to accommodate but to directly tackle the issue of what to do when we do not know the answers.

Surprise solutions

Human health epidemics are often brought to an end thanks to new awareness linked to emerging forms of knowledge, which itself brings large ramifications imbricated in many unrelated, even political, ways. Cholera and related outbreaks were the scourge of European cities at a time of peak urbanization in the 1800s. The way it was tackled in England, Paris, and Naples differed greatly, offering insight into how epidemics can be handled.

First, in England, a hard-luck approach to welfare driven by a lawyer with little sympathy for the poor, Sir Edwin Chadwick, ended up leading to major sanitation projects that put paid to many contagious diseases. His administrative approach – in marked contrast to the socially-conscious medicine championed in Germany at the time – essentially separated public health from medicine and focused on cleaning up the urban environment. No doubt aided by the industrial boom of Victorian times, it turned out that was exactly what mattered.

Meanwhile, in Paris, developments in chemistry led to a revolutionary approach to medicine and hospitals that put an end to centuries of classicism. It was, as Frank Snowden magisterially describes, a transformation in medical epistemology, not a specific medical or scientific discovery, that drove the change at a time when the city was drawing in new populations and was home to sporadic outbreaks of typhoid, pulmonary tuberculosis, and cholera. The new statistical approach allowed France's large hospital institutions to grasp the concept of contagion

– until then a folk-wisdom concept actively eschewed by professionals – and led to the major urban overhaul pioneered by George Eugene Hausmann, who for good measure introduced broad boulevards and open spaces that his political overseers also hoped would mitigate the perennial risk of revolts. The Haussman project, a slum-clearing essentially, stoked fierce resistance – and Snowden notes it shifted the locus of future outbreaks to the suburbs, a fact of some consequence in French history – but cholera never returned to the city center.

Naples, Italy's largest city at the time, didn't join the trend, and when cholera struck the city with force in 1884 its people reacted with particular shock and virulence. Stung by the experience, the authorities belatedly decided to remake the city with the sole purpose of pre-empting cholera – implementing a pure public health mandate. They turned to one of the finest epidemiologists of the time, the Bavarian scientist Max von Pettenkofer, known as the "pope of hygiene" and an expert in the prevailing medical theory about cholera at the time, which involved miasmatic groundwater vapors.

Snowden, a professor at Yale University, describes the massive *risanamento* of Naples, which involved literally raising the level of the streets, as a "cousin" of the sanitary movement in England and Paris, but with a single-minded agenda focused on the epidemic at hand. Unfortunately, the costly project ran into bankruptcy, fraud and delays, during which the principle behind the plan was eclipsed by the advent of Louis Pasteur and the germ theory of disease. Cholera returned to Naples anyway, and efforts to hide that fact to avoid social unrest led to a lasting distrust of the state.

All three of the cases above involved epidemics, although the way public health was harnessed as a paradigm differed enormously. The purest science-driven approach ended up being somewhat of a non sequitur.

In general, success in coping with endemic or pandemic human ailments comes as a result of multiple factors, some of them seemingly remote from the immediate cause at hand, as the English case shows. Professor Snowden, on that note, observes that the apparent success in using DDT to wipe out malaria in postwar Italy was for a time taken as a lesson that the same technology might be used to eradicate malaria globally, even though its success was likely achieved thanks to the "massive social uplift" of Italians' income and living conditions thanks to the Marshall Plan.

Given the shocking tendency in advanced industrial economies for obesity and diabetes to concentrate where income and living standards are weakest – exalting the penchant to buy cheaper energy-dense foods – a repetition of that today would almost certainly be the most effective way to tackle contemporary human health woes.

A natural history

Most of the sugar we eat today began its life, botanically, as a grass. Sugar cane is a perennial tall grass and its stalks are where the sucrose accumulates. Today it is the world's largest crop in terms of how much is produced, with Brazil far and away the leading source.

Probably originating on a Polynesian island, it was first domesticated in Papua New Guinea, but its commercial life is not easy there today. The island now exports coffee, cocoa and oil palm, and its people consume a vast array of wild-grown forest foods and grow yams, sharply preferring the taste of their own varieties and landraces over breeds introduced in

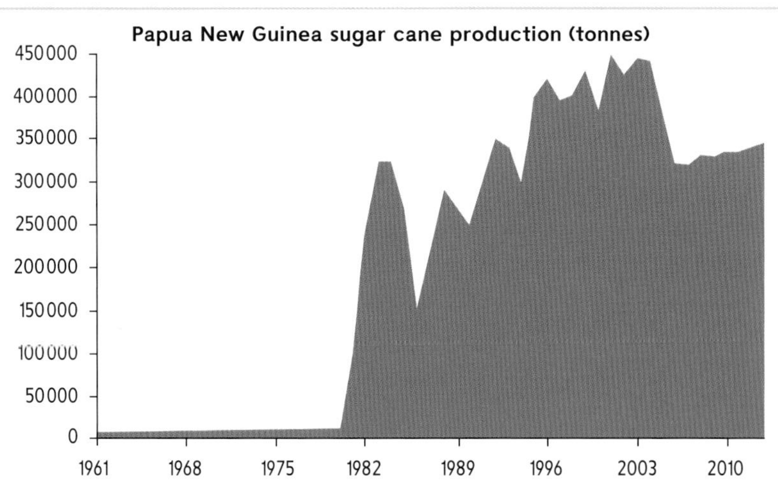

Papua New Guinea is the homeland of sugar cane, which has long been a garden crop there but never much of an industry. The nation is a net importer of sugar

Source: UN Food and Agriculture Organization

hopes of obtaining higher yields, as well as a large number of vegetables, most of them relative newcomers.

Curiously, sugar cane is not a big sector in the country – it is eighteenth in the list of food items produced by value, and the only local sugar producer, Ramu Sugar, is struggling as falling tariffs help make refined sugar the country's sixth-largest food import, according to the Food and Agriculture Organization of the United Nations - but Papua New Guinea is the spiritual home of the plant and in particular of *Saccharum officinarum,* known as "noble cane."

All quiet on the home front

This noble type is grown by subsistence farmers, who likely selected the type by watching pigs or rats, who have an unerring eye for the sweeter varieties. They grow it in gardens as it cannot survive in the wild, although a slew of its relatives thrive on the island. The global sugar cane industry is quite interested in these other kinds, in hopes they may provide some new resistance or trait suitable to where they now grow the crop in vast areas. Because Papua New Guinea is huge and considered primitive, little is known about sugar cane's biodiversity there other than that it is vast.

Commercial scientists have been collecting sugar cane germplasm specimens in Papua New Guinea since 1875, and the US Department of Agriculture joined with Australian, Hawaiian, and Dutch colonial interests to sponsor a rather famous junket that in 1928 set out in hopes of finding varieties resilient to mosaic, a virus then rampaging through Louisiana's sugar cane fields and threatening them elsewhere. The adventurous scientists collected more than 130 *officinarum* varieties and other species they named after themselves. But they appeared understandably distracted by the vast human world they encountered as they seaplaned around the eastern part of the main island. In fact, the gentleman explorers shot a lot of film and a silent black-and-white movie, *Sugar Cane Hunting by Airplane,* was made in 1929. The press seemed less interested in the biological findings than in running headlines such as "Cannibals cheated of meal by roaring seaplane motor."[18]

Sugar does have two felonies to account for. One is the cane toad introduced by its growers to Australia and now a terrifyingly successful invasive species. The other is that the mosaic virus that afflicted the

American sugar cane mutated into a new variant that attacked sorghum crops and emerged in Ohio as a serious threat to corn in the 1960s. Plant pathologists managed to develop resistant breeds in an effort that has now led to expansive use of genetically-modified varieties of corn, sparking another one of our contemporary food worries.

Way back when, sugar cane found its way to India, the presumed origin of a key constituent of the modern plant, *Saccharum spontaneum*, which has a thinner cane and produces much less sugar but is more robust and above all more resistant to diseases. That variety, quite able to live on sand dunes and along highways, is classified as a weed in many US states and in Asia is a hassle to many farmers today as it is effective in colonizing depleted agricultural soils and using dense root mats to block access to other plants.

The word "sugar," in fact, hails from Sanskrit, as does "candy," which stems from *khanda* in the same Indo-Aryan language.[19] Scribes of ancient Persia and Greece referred to "reeds that produce honey without bees." Arab traders took it to their domains in North Africa and Europe, from where it was also taken to be planted in the Canary and Madeira Islands.

There are reasons that sugar went on to become a human calorie powerhouse that are worth reviewing here, not least as the natural history has relevance going forward in a world where both the average global temperature and the human population are rising.

To grow, sugar cane needs a tropical or at least temperate climate with a lot of water and sunlight. Indeed, it is not very picky about soils and is regularly billed as the most efficient photosynthesis machine in the world. This is where sugar cane being a grass is important. Like corn and sorghum, sugar cane has a more advanced method of photosynthesis than most plants, one adopted by around half the world's grasses. Sugar cane leads its peers, too, with efficiency rates of up to seven percent in turning sunlight into chemical energy, making it a supreme food crop as well as a major contributor to carbon storage, meaning that global acreage put to sugar cane offers, relative to other foodstuffs, a kind of ecological service to mitigate climate change.

Sugar cane uses its reedy stem rather than fruit or seed structures to store photosynthate, or sucrose. The reedy structure of sugar cane stems in fact represents some fancy natural engineering, as it enables the plant – with the help of specialized bacteria – to fix atmospheric nitrogen inside its stems, skipping a strict reliance on roots as legumes and other plants do to turn atmospheric nitrogen into the ammonia they need to make proteins. This skill, known as C4 photosynthesis, not only points to sugar cane's ability to thrive in many types of soil, but also – like corn, another C4 plant that happens to be an agricultural heavyweight today and is often demonized by critics of our modern food system – highlights how a highly-evolved plant has found a way to reduce its relative reliance on the environment to produce food we can eat.

Sugar cane is in a way its own food processor. Indeed, once cut, it will spoil if not refined within hours.[20] Calling sugar a hyper-processed food is, perhaps, a compliment.

C4 photosynthesis is an evolutionary trait of some plants that allows them to thrive more than their peers with traditional C3 photosynthesis in environments that are relatively drier and hotter, which they do because they are far more efficient with water, losing only a third as much for every carbon dioxide molecule they fix. C4 grasses haven't been major players on the earth's surface very long in cosmic terms. As they need sunlight, biogeologists assume that their expansion came at the cost of dense forests, essentially creating savannas where jungles once stood.

Their emergence may have come in ebbs and flows, but the archeological record – found in the teeth of our ancestors – shows a major step change only around 6 million years ago. Their story amounts to "nature's green revolution," says Colin Osborne, a professor of plant science at the University of Sheffield and one of the foremost experts in C4 grasses and the eventual origins of agriculture.

Today, plants with the C4 pathway provide almost a third of the Earth's carbon fixation independent of the oceans – quite an achievement given that they are newcomers and have been around for only a nanosecond in the 3 billion years of photosynthetic history. Moreover, their carbon storage is six times as great as their share of planetary biomass. Only one in thirty known plant species has C4 capabilities, and yet they account for half of the plants eaten in many parts of the world today.

That, of course, is partly due to humans having cultivated them on a vast scale. Sugar cane is a C4 plant, an so are corn, sorghum, and millet, all key staples, as well as desert plants such as cactus and agave, essential foods in arid climates in the Americas. C4 plants' competitive advantage is that they are essentially very thrifty with carbon dioxide, and that's the carbon they turn into sugars. As mentioned, they also had a significant impact on landscapes, colonizing savannas, onto which hominid ancestors walked while most primates hung out in the trees.

If that sounds familiar to the story of human evolution it's because it should. The C4 story, in timing and delivery, coincides with the fateful idea of becoming bipeds and developing bigger brains. Brains are fueled uniquely by glucose, a key constituent of sugar, and C4 plants began offering a lot more of it a few million years ago.

While some animals had already taken to C4 plants, primates "stuck by the old restaurants" of leaves and fruits, says Thure Cerling, a geochemist at the University of Utah and lead researcher on a team that has just analyzed scores of archeological evidence and concluded that they show a surprise jump in grasses as dietary foods 3.5 million years ago. "Tropical grasses provided a new set of restaurants," Cerling added, noting that other primates did not follow suit.

As befits the adage that we are what we eat, teeth provided the clue. Cerling and colleagues scoured African museums to find teeth representing eleven hominid species that once roamed around Ethiopia and Kenya from 2 to 4 million years ago. Using new technologies, they drilled out tiny amounts of tooth enamel, put it in a mass spectrometer and analyzed carbon isotypes, which it is now known reveal the photosynthetic pathways used by the foods those teeth once chewed. Their findings clearly track the emergence of proto-humans who relied on C4 for the bulk of their dietary needs. This, Cerling says, requires changing the way we imagine how we obtained the added intelligence that eventually led to *Homo sapiens*.[21] Chimpanzees and gorillas stuck with their grandmothers' C3 menu and as a result their diets today are typically much high in fiber content – hence the trademark paunch of today's gorilla, who needs a lengthy lower intestine to house such food while it ferments in the gut and is broken down by microbes.

Our forebears may have had some health issues adjusting to the new ecologically abundant C4 foods, but they soldiered on and over time the extra carbons coming from C4 plant sugars allowed for them to emerge with big brains and flexible dietary skills, a combination that much later allowed us to disperse around the world to a vast array of very different and fluctuating ecosystems, each with its own food system, often in flux itself.

Adaptation was key. According to Michael Richards of the Max Planck Institute for Evolutionary Anthropology, there is some evidence that the Neanderthals in Europe relied so heavily on larger C3-fed animals that they got edged off the scene when our folks showed up with broader metabolic technologies such as the ability to eat seafood and hunt for rabbits.[22]

Around 10,000 years ago, we learned agriculture, then industrialized it, and now know more than ever before. It was only a few decades ago, for instance, that the existence of the C4 photosynthetic pathway was discovered by scientists. While the earliest undisputed C4 plant in the fossil record is a 12.5 million-year-old fossil specimen from California, ongoing research shows that what Osborne calls a "solar-powered carbon dioxide pump" led a revolutionary expansion of C4 plants more or less at the same time in the southern US Great Plains, in Argentina, Bolivia, India and Pakistan, as well as Kenya. At some point it may have accounted for 80 percent of all vegetation, far more than today, prompting many scientists to wonder about the likely environmental trigger that prompts these carbon scavengers to expand and contract – atmospheric carbon dioxide levels, global temperature shifts, forest fires, and the possibility of feedback cycles between plant and water all vie for consideration.

Osborne warns against oversimplification. He says C4 photosynthesis is likely more of a variation on a theme than a fixed trait, that its evolution owes much to contingency and that the process itself should be considered a "physiological syndrome that has evolved independently multiple times and comes in many flavors," with as many phenotypic drivers and ecological strategies.[23]

In essence, C4 was an accidental result – probably the product of a bacterial bricolage repeated many times and consisting of nabbing components from other plants – and its superior efficiency represents its relatively low investment in leaf growth, which translates into more carbon in the plant. So, while everyone agrees that people should eat more fresh fruit and vegetables, climate change means the new menu will likely be key in feeding the world. C4 plants appear better than their elder cousins at adjusting to expected conditions without producing less zinc, iron, and other critical micronutrients billions of people already don't get enough of.[24]

That's why some scientists aiming to keep the global food supply on track are racing to forcibly introduce what sugar cane has, C4 photosynthesis, to the great C3 foodstuffs, rice and wheat. The International Rice Research Institute (IRRI) in the Philippines has an entire C4 Rice Center, led by Paul Quick, working on the project, and in December 2014 announced they have already achieved a rudimentary breakthrough in a campaign aimed at boosting rice yields by 50 percent per acre.[25]

The C4 process effectively processes cheap resources such as sunlight and atmospheric nitrogen better than traditional plants, making it of obvious interest in a world of finite natural assets. For that very reason, it is very much on the mind of the biofuels sector, as the "supercharged" plants in question are also custom-built to be converted into mechanical energy.

Both maize and sugar cane are already the main players in the biofuels industry, with sugar the real star, as more than half of Brazil's huge sugar cane output goes into ethanol. Oil is old carbon, sugar cane provides new carbon, and Brazilian automobiles are kitted out with flexible-fuel motors to use the latter, a policy decision that helped drive massive expansion of sugar cane cultivation. The growth has been so big – a 52 percent increase in acreage in five years[26] – that sugar is perhaps the agricultural commodity most sensitive to the price of oil, which is both a farm input and a competitor product. The recent decline in oil prices has pushed sugar's wholesale international price down by almost half since 2011, but it is still twice as high as 2002, according to the food price index of FAO, the United Nations agency.

Brazil's got cane

Year	Sugar production		Sugar exports		Ethanol production	
	Brazil	World	Brazil	World	Brazil	World
1990	8.0	110.8	1.6	28.4	12	20
2000	16.5	130.0	6.5	36.5	11	30
2005	28.1	140.7	18.4	48.0	16	46
2010	38.0	156.7	27.5	55.5	27.5	103
2015/16*	38.0	178.7	26.5	63.8	29.8	n/a

Brazil accounted for two-thirds of the increase in global sugar production and almost all global exports from 1990 through 2010. Production and export figures in millions of tonnes, while ethanol figure is in billions of liters

*Forecast

Source: International Sugar Organization

The price signal

Year	All food	Sugar
1990	178.1	107.2
1991	127.2	105.0
1992	128.5	109.2
1993	142.2	105.5
1994	171.9	110.3
1995	188.5	125.3
1996	169.7	131.1
1997	161.4	120.3
1998	126.6	108.6
1999	89.0	93.2
2000	116.1	91.1
2001	122.6	94.6
2002	97.8	89.6
2003	100.6	97.7
2004	101.7	112.7
2005	140.3	118.0
2006	209.6	127.2
2007	143.0	161.4
2008	181.6	201.4
2009	257.3	160.3
2010	302.0	188.0
2011	368.9	229.9
2012	305.7	213.3
2013	251.0	209.8
2014	241.2	201.8
2015	197.5	172.4

Sugar prices fell less than other commodity prices in the 1990s, rose less in the 2000-2010 period, and have declined less since. The chart shows price trends as measured by the FAO Food Price Index, a trade-weighted index that tracks prices on international markets of major food commodity groups. Domestic sugar prices can vary substantially from FAO's index due to national market rules reflecting the historic desire for self-sufficiency in sugar. The graph uses annual unadjusted prices to smooth out seasonal swings

Source: United Nations Food and Agriculture Organization

Alas, it turns out that innovative work in biology is concerned that the photosynthetic advantage of tall grasses such as sugar cane would erode if the amount of carbon dioxide in the atmosphere rose to 700 parts per million. After all, while the C4 plants can take the heat, they evolved to deal with relative carbon dioxide starvation. As some say carbon dioxide levels may plausibly hit the 700 level by the end of the century, it's quite a concern. Xin-Guang Zhu and his research partner suggest that efficiency could still be restored – and the world's population fed – but it would require modifications to plants' canopy structure, basically making grasses leafier, leaving less carbon to be stored as sucrose!

On its own, sugar cane flowers only irregularly, a process that can take up to three months and distracts the plant from growing a longer stalk to store sugar.[27] Growers try to dissuade it, even breeding for non-flowering types, although that also clashes with the tendency to generate new varieties, which means that resilience will likely require more trips to Papua New Guinea.

On a brighter note, if C4 plants do lose market share in the biosphere due to global warming, farmers can at least worry less about crabgrass and other weeds – they, too are C4 plants – and try to grow more fresh produce![28]

Surprise!

As this book aims to explore the public health concerns about sugar in the human diet, it is inevitable that a broad notion of what constitutes public health be entertained. After all, if drastically reducing sugar supply leads to a calorie shortfall and growing more nutrient-rich food crops turns out to be harder than expected, the applause for the anti-sugar mission may not be deafening.

On that note, consider the recent findings of Francisco Mello of the University of Sao Paulo. He set out to answer the question about land use and sugar cane ethanol, taking soil samples up to one meter below the surface at more than 100 field sites to assess whether the new crop is a carbon debtor or creditor to what came before. He found that planting sugar cane on the *cerrado*, or savannah lands, led to a 26 percent decline in carbon stocks on the land. Where sugar cane replaced former pastures, the loss was 10 percent although variation was large, reflecting historical usage patterns. Meanwhile, sugar cane resulted in net carbon

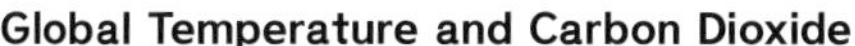

Global Temperature and Carbon Dioxide

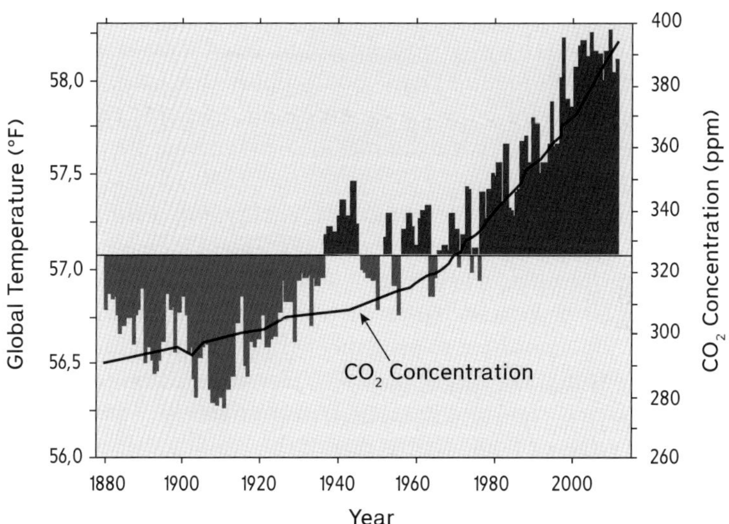

The carbon dioxide concentration in the earth's atmosphere has risen by almost 50 percent since Matthew Arnold's time as indicated by the sloping line above. The bars represent years when temperatures were above or below the long-term average. C4 plants can handle the heat but were designed to thrive with lower levels of carbon

Source: U.S. Global Change Research Program

gains for soils formerly under cultivation for annual crops. The upshot, bluntly, is that those who want to slow climate change might need to go easy on the vegetables and load up on sugar, and now and then a steak. Once again, the reason for that is that sugar's biological source is one of nature's green revolutionaries. While sugar cane may be complex in evolutionary and physiological terms, its product is exceptionally simple and flexible.

Simplicity and flexibility are incredible assets. That said, they need to be handled with care in complex systems, which tend to be more robust when home to specialists rather than generalists. A surprisingly strong view on this comes from none other than Karl Marx, who, writing in *Capital* about the rise of a new form of industrial capitalism in Europe and using the new language coming from biology and chemistry, referred to an "irreparable rift in the interdependent process of social metabolism, a metabolism prescribed by the natural laws of life itself."[29] He referred to ineluctably social processes, most notably intense urbanization, which required new food supplies that upset soil fertility, the ultimate source of nutrition. Interestingly, even his version of the rational governance of the human metabolism with nature invoked "the least expenditure of energy."

In human digestion, spending less energy but eating the same amount is likely to lead to weight problems. Energy dynamics are slightly different in practice, though, as it is easier for production and consumption to be dislocated. That's increasingly the case with the food system too. While it is hard to get a nicely ripe tomato in New York, and virtually impossible not to get one in Naples, major commodity staples such as sugar and the starchy crops transport nicely – after being refined into crystals or flour. That is one of the reasons that rural frontier Americans were big sugar buyers, and why Nepal was keen on sugar after the quake.

Compared to renewable energy sources such as wind or solar, one of the great attractions of biofuels is the flexibility they offer because they can take liquid form, thus making them, like oil, easy to ship long distances. The attraction of such mobile fuels is, of course, entirely a product of social arrangements, with all their attendant conceits and deceits.

The same is true of much of what is happening in the effort to develop so-called third generation biofuels. One of the most pure-science pursuits happening today, this is geared to finding a way to go beyond the soluble sugars and starch stored in plant biomass and tap the plants' cell walls directly, which house structural polysaccharides, the mother lode of carbohydrates and not part of our food system at all.

The basic idea is to harvest the food, then process the residual plant debris. Sugar cane and its C4 colleagues – notably maize and sorghum, but also some grasses – are once again the target of research finding a way to do this without applying so much heat and pressure, and so many chemicals that efficiency gains drift away. Breakthroughs are likely to occur as with the C4 rice project, by toggling the gene code to reduce the natural resistance of plant cell walls – related to the plants' will to live as discrete entities – to enzymatic deconstruction.[30]

Progress will likely be made faster according to human factors beyond the sheer merits of the relative plants, say researchers at Wageningen University, one of the world's leading agricultural research institutes. Sugar cane has a very complex genome, making it a greater challenge. Even more relevantly, deliberate genetic changes can be triggered faster in annual crops like maize and sorghum.

So there's a need for speed – but it's not in the objective nature of things, lying rather in what Marx alluded to as a broader metabolism.

Slouching into the modern era

The human body extracts sugars from all food for its use, and as noted we have had millions of years to grow accustomed to C4 plants that produce such chemical energy more efficiently.

What we did not have was refined sugar on an industrial scale. While Alexander the Great noted that India was producing sugar crystals 2,000 years ago, western societies were not really in the loop until crusaders noticed the widespread use of sweets in the Muslim world. They tried to grow the plant in Europe but the climate was for the most part too temperate, and limited sugar supplies meant that for centuries it functioned only as a rare spice available only to the elite.

That reflects geography. In fact, a typical American diet today is split about evenly between C3 and C4 plants, according to Cerling. The former comprises vegetables, fruits, and grains such as wheat, oats, rye, and barley, while the latter comes largely from corn and sorghum – much of which is eaten by animals before humans.

While wheat has higher protein content than corn, and is a C3 plant presumably familiar to cows of European extraction, it is not used much with North American cattle, who today are mostly Holsteins and mainly eat corn in feedlots. While wheat has a higher protein content than corn, and is roughly similar in terms of energy, cows tend to eat less of it, slowing their growth, and when they do eat it many experience bovine bloating due to the more rapid fermentation of wheat starches.

American nutritional science was in a sense founded on what to feed cattle. In a famous experiment conducted in Wisconsin before World War I, Stephen Babcock, armed with a doctorate in agricultural chemistry earned in Germany, was granted permission to carry out the "single-grain experiment" to see how cows fared if they ate only one type of grain. His aim was to do a randomized controlled trial to determine what the optimal dietary balance of carbohydrates, protein, and fats was for cows, as hitherto he had been able only to investigate their manure in what is known as an observational study.

In the first trial, an oat-fed cow promptly died and Babcock's superiors insisted he stop. But he managed to get another chance and, working with Edwin B. Hart, it was agreed to run trials wherein heifers ate only corn, only bran, only wheat, while a control set ate a mixed diet. The corn-fed cows fared best, while the calves of the wheat-fed animals were stillborn.

Babcock and Hart concluded that there must be micronutrients beyond the three main dietary categories that made a digestive difference. A year after their work was done, Casimir Funk, a Polish biochemist working in London, coined the word "vitamine." A slew of discoveries then ensued, some even going back in time, leading to the realization that vitamin deficiencies were behind a raft of diseases at the time, including scurvy, pellagra, beriberi, and rickets. Eventually, Nobel Prizes were doled out.

Meanwhile, much of Europe has in fact had a C3 menu. That makes sense given the region's relatively cool temperatures, but very likely also represented cultural preferences – and probably power relations, too, in cases where some parts of society had restricted access to foods. In Italy, bones of people who lived in Bronze Age settlements revealed that they apparently ate a domestic millet, as they score positively for C4 traces. But further south in "The Boot" – in the homeland of the Mediterranean diet – C4 was off the table, and people ate mostly wheat and barley, with only low levels of animal protein.

In what is now Croatia, next to northern Italy, carbon and nitrogen isotypes show no C4 traces at all during Antiquity, and people began eating fish only after the Roman conquest. Then there was a curious switch in the Middle Ages, with fish dropping off the menu, replaced by C4 millet. Archeologists see this as the sign of a large-scale cultural change, likely due to the wholesale invasion of the region by Slavic peoples around that time.[31]

Archeologists have also looked for carbon traces of the diet in late medieval Spain, choosing human bones buried near Gandia on the coast south of Valencia where both Christians and Muslims lived side by side from the thirteenth to the sixteenth centuries. This is a particularly fascinating data set as the period spans the time when the Islamic rule of al-Andalus gradually gave way to the Riconquista in the region, turning once-dominant Muslims into *mudejares* and, after the royal decree forbidding Islamic practice, *moriscos*, who are widely understood to have quietly continued with their faith.

The Muslims, with a millennial tradition in making marzipan and other sweets, had brought sugar cane to cultivate in the area in the eighth century, and the tradition in Gandia was to grow it as a secondary crop, mill it with a small animal-powered *trapig* or distribute the cane as a pleasure for kids and adults. That changed with the Riconquista. Once ensconced in power, the local Duke of Gandia took ownership of all the land, had a refining mill built and ordered the Muslims to grow more sugar cane as a cash crop for export, using the proceeds to import more cheaply-grown wheat from elsewhere in Spain. One of the world's first confectionery cookbooks was shortly thereafter produced in Barcelona.

Interestingly, the isotopes showed that the Muslims of Gandia, buried facing Mecca, had far more C4 traces than their Christian neighbors.[32] It seems they chewed sugar cane and their labor was compensated with sorghum, a grain long recognized by Islamic dietaries[33] but spurned by Christians, while the Christians ate imported wheat paid for by sugar exports. The evident hierarchical segregation was then exacerbated when the Spanish monarch outlawed *hala'l* butchering practices – making protein harder to get. Shortly thereafter Spain's Muslims were sent into exile – more or less just as sugar cane production began ramping up in Brazil.

The pace quickens

Around this time diabetes appeared to be making a splash in London. One of the staples of the literature on the origins of diabetes dates from 1674, when Thomas Willis wrote *Pharmaceutice rationalis*, a text in which he christened the disorder with the name *diabetes mellitus*, using the Latin word for honey and noting that those who suffered from it also had urine that tasted "wonderfully sweet, as if it were imbued with honey or sugar."

His analogy has had remarkable, perhaps devastating staying power.

The observation had in fact been made before, inscribed on Egyptian papyri in 1,500 BCE and astutely observed by Susruta, an Indian physician in the sixth century who used the image of honey urine and noted the illness appeared to affect people who ate a lot of rice, cereals, and sweets, while a contemporary Chinese doctor was already advising afflicted patients to avoid sex and liquor.

The word "diabetes" was coined by Demetrius of Apameia in the first century, and shortly thereafter a Greek peer living in Cappadocccia, Aretaus, gave a clinical description of the illness, noting it was chronic in nature and consisted of a "melting down of the flesh and limbs into urine."[34] Given the global recording of sweet-tasting urine, starting almost 5,000 years ago, one might conclude that sugar must be the toxic cause. But if so, where did they get the sugar?

Despite great fascination with sugar, average consumption in Britain was still around four pounds per head in 1700, a generation after Willis wrote, according to Sidney Mintz,[35] the outstanding chronicler of the subject. By 1800 it had risen to 18 pounds. That's rather less than the 90 pounds it reached a century later.

Willis, who reportedly recommended beating epileptics with a stick as a cure, not punishment, most likely saw the signs of dramatic social change, including in diets. England had been prospering, and in the century before his observation the average real income of a London laborer had risen by more than 50 percent compared to the cost of food. Above all that meant more beef, the consumption of which was a point of pride for the British. But the boom was just about to enter a long stage of decline, dropping by a quarter when measured against the cost of subsistence victuals.[36]

Undernutrition spread as the riches of trade did not reach every household. It was after all the beginning of a world-changing period of colonial exchanges, which surely represented a regime change in social, ecological, and dietary practices in Britain and elsewhere in Europe, just as globalization is rapidly altering those same systems today. Diabetes and diet problems reflected a metabolic shock and, as will be shown later, London had all the characteristics now emerging in developing countries, where urbanization is happening at a faster pace than anywhere ever before.

Affordable sugar for the masses was still some way off. Health problems at the time reflected other social strains, especially as hard-core industrialization and its corollary Poor Laws and urban infectious disease came later. In the 1700s, English society was perhaps like the USA or Britain of the past few decades, with financial speculation (the South Sea Bubble stock-market crash), people migrating from the country to the city, a new cash economy (income inequality), a wave of exploitation in the form of slavery affecting other people but the cause of apprehension (refugees), the rise of new expressive forms like the novel (the internet), and falling real wages. There was also an inordinate amount of barley-based gin (binge drinking), which would even be replaced by coffee and tea (energy drinks marketed as performance-enhancing for sports), always to substitute London's noxious water.

Andrew Hogarth, the popular printmaker who apparently became a beef-eating militant after a trip to the "effeminate" Mediterranean countries, depicted all this change with some early examples of dietary moralism. With his famous incisions of *Beer Street* and *Gin Lane*, he decried the

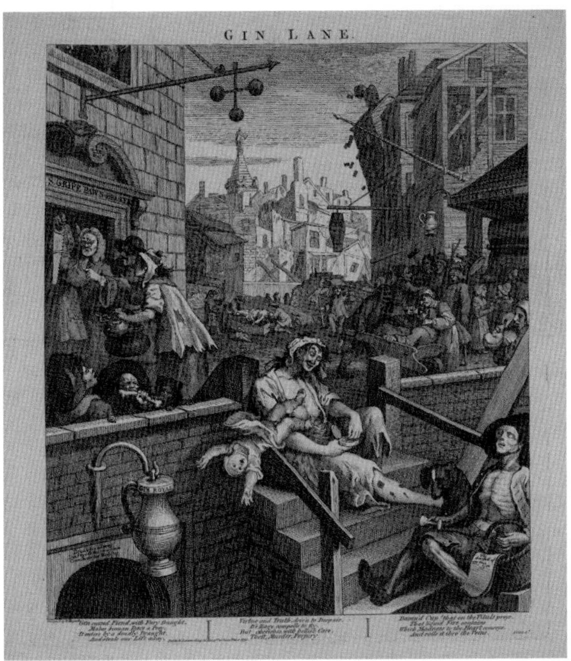

Andrew Hogarth's *Gin Lane*. Hogarth's print was part of a set; the other, "Beer Street," depicted happy workers in contrast to the ravages of the gin drinkers

so-called "gin epidemic" as leading to dissolute people killing their own babies, while promoting drinking beer as the slow road to prosperity.

Sascha Muldoon, a British doctor, sees the artist's work as an early and admirable example of public health advocacy. "What we need is a modern day Hogarth," she wrote in a sympathetic analysis wherein she noted that the prints also show how dreadful the Gin Lane environment really was, noting signs of contagious disease, a snail, and a possible suicide attempt in the background of the scene, as well as suggesting that the breast-feeding woman taking snuff as her infant falls into a river may be an example of the pitfalls of what happens when the poor try to emulate the habits of the affluent.[37] Epidemiologists always say that social factors are important, and Muldoon is more forceful than most medical practitioners in emphasizing this. Still, her assumption is that there is a problem – alcoholism on Gin Lane, and again in modern Britain today in her view – that needs to be fixed and the question is what kind of regulatory approach should be adopted.

This is an instructive case. Hogarth was in fact championing the Gin Act, a parliamentary law introduced in 1751 that sought drastically to curtail gin consumption by restricting wholesale trade in the spirit. Gin was at the time a relatively new entry in London's menu and had proven a smash hit, with per capita consumption in 1741 some ten times higher than it is today. But the Gin Act, formerly the Sale of Spirits Act, was not deliberated as a public health measure. Quite the contrary. It was passed in the wake of a perceived burglary spree, and the criminals in question hailed from the "dregs" of society "aspiring still to a degree beyond that which belongs to them." That was the phrase used by Henry Fielding, the author of *Tom Jones,* who wrote a lengthy pamphlet full of allusions to ancient Greece and Rome about the "causes of the increases of robbers" and offering "proposals for remedying this growing evil" that had affluent people afraid to go outside.

It is an extraordinary document of elite folklore and social epidemiology.[38] Fielding defines a broader cause of the problem, which he sees as a change in a natural feudal social ranking system, and a disease vector, which is the proliferation of "luxury" brought by external trade. This latter appeals to low-ranking human subjects, who due to "greatly changed Customs, Manners and Habits" no longer feel bound to be loyal to the social hierarchy above them, and triggers temptation to increase consumption even while cutting back on exertion. From such a mix inevitably emerge some who become skilled thieves.

Fielding then posits a collective goal which is that people should reject idleness and engage in "busyness" to boost national wealth, which shall not be spent on unnecessary items such as entertainment, drink, and gambling. Warning of the risk of contagious "plague," he admonishes upper-class people for the "moral evil" of their luxuries while saying that lower-class people tempted by expensive diversions are committing "political evil." He then notes that taxation won't work to suppress gin – which he sees as a symptom rather than a catalyst of disorder – because as it happens past efforts to levy it had been undermined by corrupt local tyrants. His remedy, then, is simply to ban the sale of gin in all bars and establishments other than those visited by the affluent classes, as such establishments are characterized by "decency."

In short, in a nineteenth-century version of champagne socialism, his apparent initial recognition of the environmental factors ailing the less privileged withers away in his final policy formulation. Fielding also appeared to be willing to abandon one of his original premises – that "in free countries, at least, it is a branch of liberty claimed by the people to be as wicked and profligate as their superiors."

Readers are of course free to make whatever political observations they like about Fielding's positions. It should also be noted that he went on to propose a kind of welfare reform, more or less a levy on everyone to guarantee a basic income for the poor, who in exchange would be compelled to work or jailed. He articulated a modern argument, weaving together regulation, taxation, and even a six-day work week in exchange for benefits.

The "gin epidemic" triggered early fumbling efforts to formulate a public health policy, and they show how vested interests are hard at work. Fielding tried to square the circle – cut the naughty pleasure, offer some consolation – in ways acceptable to his peer group. While not quite Marie Antoinette dismissing the poor with her apocryphal "let them eat cake," such interventions often amount to a "cut the sugar and add some starch" formula that may not solve a problem that hasn't been fully understood.

Assessing the merits of the case for public order to justify the Gin Act would require knowing the real scale of the crime wave that allegedly took place at a late phase of the so-called gin epidemic. It turns out that the murder rate was 100 times less than in Rome at the time, and also that the broader property crime rate increased later in the century – after gin had fallen out of favor.[39] The so-called gin epidemic appears to be what Paul Campos calls a moral panic.

The most popular print Hogarth made, as it happens, was *Midnight Modern Conversation*, depicting eleven well-dressed and well-fed men laughing around a table in a well-appointed salon. No fewer than 23 empty wine bottles and a grandfather clock indicating it is four o'clock in the morning can be seen.

To take the social factors cited by public health officials seriously, we do not need another Hogarth behind a lobbying campaign, but to look out for snails.

Gin had muscled beer off of Britain's drinking menu at the time, and the government did not at all mind as it was a market for surplus grains and a new source of tax revenue, especially as it had just banned French wine imports. Gin turned out to be a hit, especially among the poorer people in London, many of them recent residents of villages with tight-knit systems of mutual social monitoring, but now making a shift in anonymous and squalid slum housing and facing rising food costs. Gin also provided calories at a relatively low cost, lower than beer, at a time of high and volatile food and basic grain prices.[40]

London had grown tenfold in two centuries to reach a population of half a million in 1700, buoyed by a booming wool trade and high real wages by European standards at the time. But that reversed in the 1700s, and squalid living conditions and appalling infant mortality became the norm. Deaths outnumbered baptisms in the 1700s, and the city only grew thanks to even more migration from the countryside after laws closed off access to public lands.

"The gin epidemic did not occur in a vacuum," says Ernest Abel, a professor at Wayne State University in Detroit and an expert on alcohol and drug-related health issues. His research interests led him to scour archives for signs that Fielding and Hogarth might have had inklings about fetal alcohol syndrome. He found they were mostly spouting Whiggish hearsay, and even discovered that the artist had engaged in an early form of media spin with his claim to have charitably produced low-cost copies of *Gin Street* to popularize the message among the poor, as the price was far above what people facing daily food insecurity could afford.

Finding a job, unsurprisingly, was apparently not difficult. Fielding in fact closes his 240-page pamphlet with a curious letter "to the public" lamenting "the rude behavior and insolence of servants of all kinds." Not only were they uppity, but the sanction of firing them proved ineffective as "they find no manner of difficulty" in finding jobs elsewhere. Meanwhile, well-off women in London at the time frequently hired newly-arrived migrants as wet nurses, and these would quite likely use sweetened liquor to pacify the infants they cared for, according to Abel, who sees social factors as more than simple income levels to acknowledge and ignore.

Even soldiers and sailors were less than fighting fit due to knocking back gin, according to an anonymous 1736 broadside addressed to the House of Commons.[41] The epidemic was serious because the gin drinkers were all likely to die young and "deprive the landowners of a work force which in turn would result in higher wages," scolded Adam Holden in another tome published that year that evoked damage done to health, lives, trade, manufacture "and the landed interests of this island." Holden, like Hogarth, advocated beer, not only because it was a traditional British drink but because "an honest man may smoak [*sic*] a pipe or two of tobacco with a pint or two of good beer for a whole evening, but is so suddenly demolish'd by the force of tyrant gin that he has scarcely time to puff out half a dozen whiffs."

Not everyone had such a narrow view of the public interest, of course. Some pamphleteers campaigned in favor of gin, or at least against the "scandalous libel" of the government's proposed crackdown. Drinking is a ubiquitous practice, while low wages create social problems, one of them wrote in 1736. And anyway, intoxication by gin is no different than by beer, he said, adding that most of the highwaymen of the time seemed to be wine drinkers – code at the time for affluence.[42]

Further evidence that policy-makers of the day had ulterior agendas comes from America. Early colonial settlers held alcohol in high regard, often drinking wine with sugar for breakfast, cider or beer for lunch, and toddies after work. Alcohol was considered medicinal and also conducive to social health, so was amply poured at barn-raisings and militia musterings to foster reciprocity and trust. Hired hands drank with their bosses.[43]

According to Jessica Warner, a professor at the University of Toronto who worked for a long time with the city's mental health and addiction center, the gin epidemic is an example of how the public health model often ends up being harnessed to a moralistic crusade invariably targeting the working poor. Her historical verdict? Replete with an urban backdrop, an underclass, and images of failed mothers, "it was in many ways Europe's first drug scare."

The campaign to stamp out gin in the 1700s had, as we have just seen, no real health content at all. In a template of how many campaigns are perceived today, it was entirely driven by economic concerns and elite interests. Moreover, today the utility of scare tactics is often more imaginary than real, as underscored by a recent Swiss study showing that young men who smoke cigarettes or marijuana, or drink alcohol, tend to seek out more information about health and risk factors related to substance abuse than their abstaining peers, and are also better able to understand it when they find it.[44]

That is clearly both an opportunity and a challenge for public health professionals. However, moralizing and even disgust-based tactics oddly remain in vogue for many in the policy sphere, as exemplified by New York City Health Commission's decision to release "Man drinking fat" in a 2009 anti-obesity campaign. The video, which has been seen more than a million times, shows a seemingly slim man pour himself a can of globby fat and then slurp it down somewhat messily. It ends with an appeal to "cut out" soda and other sugary drinks and claims that "one can a day can make you 10 pounds fatter every year." As soda drinks obviously contain no fat, the decision to run the video represented a clear political strategy based on a "major gross-out factor." Emails obtained by *The New York Times* under the state Freedom of Information law revealed an internal discussion at the Health Commission in which the chief nutritionist warned that the message was "absurd," but health commissioner Thomas Farley insisted on leveraging what he described as people's "fear" of becoming fat and a third official in charge of media and marketing insisted that the key thing was for the message to go "viral." A compromise was found centering on the word "can."

Three years later, Dr. Farley unveiled the *Take Care New York 2012* report, which stated that sugary drinks are the source of half the extra 250 calories the city's residents eat each day compared to thirty years ago. Its source was a paper by Eric A. Finkelstein, a professor at Duke University's campus in Singapore with a penchant for economic analyses, who in 2013 calculated that a 20 percent tax on sugar-sweetened beverages would probably lead to weight loss of 1.6 pounds in the first year and 2.9 pounds in the long run. In 2014, he ran a more sophisticated model, calibrated to incomes and likely substitution effects, and found that an even higher 26 percent tax on sugary drinks would lead to a low-income person, assumed to drink more soda, to lose half a pound in one year and 1.5 pounds over a decade. Weight losses by higher-income people would be half that amount.[45]

That's a far cry from 10 pounds every year![46]

While evidently it could be argued that weight loss might require increased physical exercise or removal of environmental toxins that may trigger obesity already in the womb, the exercise here has been to stick with the hymn book of focusing on cutting out, by choice or through the tax code, sugary drinks. The main reason the predicted weight loss is lower is due to substitution effects, meaning people would offset their foregone carbohydrates by consuming more salt and fats. Communications strategists generally cut that part. Increasingly the YouTube jingle resembles another viral media icon, Hogarth's *Gin Lane.*

Jessica Warner ran the numbers on that historical episode, which represented one of the first times a modern government invoked an epidemic to regulate distribution and sales of a good. Scouring parliamentary and excise records, she found overall duties on gin rose 1,200 percent from 1700 to 1771. However, taxes were often eluded and when lawmakers aimed at directly curbing retail distribution they provoked an open revolt that transformed "a simple indulgence into an act of political protest" and prompted thousands of shops and distillers to rebrand their evasive concoctions "parliament brandy." The populace is pleased to see real crimes punished but feels alienated and oppressed when regulations target "actions which are thought neither pernicious nor scandal," mused an editorial in one London newspaper.

Meanwhile, the various interventions caused sporadic short-lived declines but did not stop steadily increasing consumption. Per capita consumption of spirits rose almost fourfold in the first three decades of the century, then dropped 24 percent in a year due to a new tax law, then grew again by 60 percent in six years, according to Warner. But here's the rub: peak consumption actually occurred in 1743, and had already fallen by 20 percent when Fielding wrote about robbers and insolent servants. The controversy around the Gin Act ended up being a non-event as, remarkably, consumption continued to plummet and by the end of the 1760s had fallen by two-thirds as people literally grew bored with it. The regulatory ineptitude would shortly be repeated with beverage taxes that outraged colonists on the other side of the Atlantic.

3 The Rap Sheet

I hesitate not to declare, no matter how sorely I shall wound our vanity, that so gross is our ignorance of the real nature of the physiological disorders, called diseases, that it would perhaps be better to do nothing, and resign the complaint we are called upon to treat to the resources of nature, than to act as we are frequently compelled to do, without knowing the why and the wherefour of our conduct, and at obvious risk of hastening the end of the patient.

François Magendie

Sugar is a sweet nothing, nutritionally, but works wonders on our taste buds and packs a lot of energy. How did it attract the ire of the food police? A few key facts lurk behind the trend, which warrant inspection.

First, people weigh more, and the corpulence that began gathering pace in western societies is making inroads into countries traditionally associated with poverty and malnutrition. Second, it has become fashionable, certainly among the comfortable classes, to worry about processed and pre-made foods, which are staking out an ever-larger share of what we eat and are often juiced up with sugar to facilitate shelf life and enhance flavor. Third, officialdom has decided it was wrong to promulgate guidelines indicating that fats, often eaten sprinkled with salt, were the cause of human adiposity, leaving an explanatory void. Fourth, extraordinary medical successes in stamping out contagious diseases whetted both the desire to find new health problems to cure and the appetite to identify their etiological cause. Fifth, laboratory rodents that eat a lot of extra sugar almost invariably pack it on.

All of these things are true and conspire to put sugar in the judicial dock.

On the first count, while obesity seems to be plateauing in rich countries, it is rising in developing nations. This is primarily occurring in cities where urbanization is occurring at unprecedented speed. Higher cash incomes and the dense population networks of cities present new menus that are typically higher in energy and starchiness, and lower in nutrients and foliage. Sometimes called "coca-colonization," this local variant of globalization often flings people who formerly had subsistence lifestyles suddenly into an everyday social system with higher calorie counts and completely different physical routines than their former rural homes.

On the second charge, many people on the happier side of the growing economic and educational inequalities in already-urbanized western societies are clearly using their discretion to seek out closer personal ties to nature and can afford to see beyond the "cheap food" that helped trigger the Industrial Revolution and consequent prosperity. Coca-Cola sales are falling, kale sales are rising, and if you want there are now organic Cheetos.

Thirdly, the administrative reach of governmental functions has expanded with modernity, and with that public health has become more autonomous from the age-old tradition of medicine. Professionals tasked with this function are expected to identify trends on an abstract level – often scanning scientific knowledge to model risk factors rather than relying on the expensive and fragmented world of therapeutic casework – and then broker the needs of multiple interest groups to formulate pre-emptive regulations. Doctors remain busy but can lean on the Hippocratic Oath – "first, do no harm" – whereas inaction by public health officials is perceived as failure or a sign of irrelevance.

Fourth, there is understandable frustration that, in a world that celebrates abundances and has largely triumphed over diseases that once snatched young lives with appalling regularity, chronic illnesses – obesity is often linked to a suite of cardiovascular ailments in turn linked to excessive inflammation of our vital organs – persist and even proliferate.

On the fifth count, well, laboratory rats have been assigned a niche in the scientific ecosystem because they allow what humans do not – to run large numbers of randomized trials hinging on single factors in relatively short time frames. That's invaluable, although there are potentially limitless factors to test and there is inevitably a shadow of doubt about what we might call the laboratory rat's socioeconomic status.

Heavy talk about the food system

Sugar consumption has never been as high as in our era. In 1900, humans consumed around 8 million tonnes of sugar. Since then the population has risen by almost fivefold, while sugar consumption rose twice as fast. In the past decade, it has grown fastest in Asia, Africa, and the Middle East.[1]

At the same time, waistlines are expanding almost everywhere.

Indeed, if current trends continue, a stunning 86 percent of Americans will be overweight or obese by 2030, and by 2048 every single one will be. By 2102 none will be merely overweight, according to calculations published in the academic journal of The Obesity Society, an advocacy group primarily funded by pharmaceutical companies.[2]

Iconic headlines are churned out claiming ours is the first generation that will not live longer than its predecessor. Severe obesity can knock up to twenty years off an individual's lifespan, and the current trend will reduce average longevity by almost a year – an effect larger than all accidental deaths combined – according to the banner story the prestigious *New England Journal of Medicine* published in 2005. They add that the figure may rise to up to five years as people are becoming obese at a younger age.[3] "The U.S. population may be inadvertently saving Social Security by becoming obese," the ten authors wryly observe.

Such claims have an illustrious history. The *Ramayana,* written in India at around the time Plato was holding his symposia in Athens, observed that "in the Golden Age, people lived on fruits and roots that were obtained without any labor," but that "the lifespan of people became shortened" as a result of agriculture, described as a sin.[4]

It's de rigeur to describe obesity as having "multifactorial" causes and tick off sedentary behavior, education, tobacco and alcohol, and a generally "obesogenic" environment full of advertising and video screens, but food is invariably seen as the prime culprit for fatness. As fat has recently been exonerated from that status after a lengthy run, it's now sugar, distributed through snacks and soft drinks, but also via canned soup and even artisanal dried meat in picturesque villages in the Alps. Meanwhile, even more sugar is produced than those consumption figures represent — much goes on ethanol — signaling that there's no looming shortage and raising the thorny question as to how much is actually eaten.

Acknowledging that limit while using the best data available and attempting to control for a suite of variables including ageing, urbanization, income, and even levels of physical exercise and alcohol use, Dr. Lustig and a team of researchers at Stanford University ran a massive global test and found a link between how much sugar is available and diabetes prevalence. Per capita sugar supply to the global food system has risen almost a third to 280 calories a day, far above the American Heart Association's recommended upper daily limit of 150 calories for and adult man and 100 for a woman. Every can of soda – or 150 calories per person per day – translated into a 1.1 percent increase in the likelihood of diabetes, they found in their stark but methodologically savvy study published in 2013.[5]

The study explicitly touted both sugar's link to diabetes and at the same time downplayed any link to obesity, keying in on public fear of disease and suggesting there is something uniquely problematic about sugar rather than overeating in general. In line with that, public health policies must aim to reduce its consumption rather than promote increased physical activity or other measures.

That is the line endorsed by Action on Sugar, a UK advocacy group that enthusiastically cites the study in presentations calling sugar "the new tobacco." It calls for hefty taxes, advertising bans and rules obliging food manufacturers to reformulate their products with less sugar content. The lobby's scientific director, Dr. Aseem Malholtra, described Dr. Lustig's study as showing sugar had a tenfold correlation to diabetes rates and thus constitutes causal proof of a connection.

Meanwhile, Sugar Nutrition, a UK group that describes itself as a network of evidence-based nutritionists but whose website is reticent about any financial sponsorship, emphasized that causality was precisely what the study did *not* show, by its authors' own admission, as it did not outline a mechanism for sugar to trigger diabetes – whose prevalence has doubled in the UK in the past decade despite sugar consumption dropping by 6 percent. It added rather wanly that more sugary foods may be wasted than the analysis assumed.

Welcome to the battle! Neither of the opposing lobbies noted that the study itself identified anomalous countries where diabetes is frequent but obesity is not, such as the Philippines, France, and Sri Lanka, where diabetes quadrupled in a decade while obesity remained virtually absent, or the opposite, such as New Zealand, where diabetes remained nearly even as obesity rose. Nor did either side zero in on the empirical gem buried in the study itself: when sugar was calculated as a fraction of total food calories rather than in terms of availability, a one percent increase in the former shrank the correlation with diabetes prevalence to 0.167 percent.

Sugar science is driven by parties with consistent policy agendas. Those who want a crackdown regularly invoke the specter of "Big Food" even though the global sugar market is worth about as much as insurance fraud in the USA and has less than half the turnover of a large automobile company. Multinational companies are "manufacturing epidemics" by forcing poor consumers to buy unhealthy packaged foods, says the lead author of the aforementioned study, who wants a new discipline of "corporatology" to examine how they can be reined in.[6]

That sounds like a fashionable narrative. And that's often the destiny of smart, well-meaning and even thorough studies based on correlation: like sugar itself, they excel at offering an excited overview, commendably generating public interest, but just when you are done with the "sugar rush" and could use some micronutrients they blame the hoary icon of greedy businesses.

A more material history might be useful. Many people recall that foods can be adulterated with real toxins, and may look to brands as guarantors of safety. One can build an argument with equal force on social inequalities being more central to disease vectors.

A survey of adults in Finland found that metabolic syndrome afflicted those with nine years of schooling precisely twice as often as those with a university degree, and this held true even after adjusting for myriad confounding factors including smoking, drinking, exercise, marital status, and even the amount of vegetables and berries people ate. The "education gradient" could not be explained away by any behavioral factor, not even height, which could be a proxy for malnutrition as a youth. Amazingly, lower education was an autonomous metabolic marker as far as the public health system was concerned. The authors suggested that "more research is needed" on how such a purely social factor could appear such a powerful mediator of a medical condition.[7]

Educational level is not the only channel through which our human relations can generate disease. Stress on the job is another. The now legendary Whitehall Study of more than 10,000 civil servants in London, aged 35 to 55, also found that metabolic syndrome was twice as likely for those who suffered stress at work. Incredibly, employees suffering on-the-job stress and given lower latitude to perform their tasks were more likely to have a BMI above 30 than their seniors who did not, and this held true at every point along the spectrum, even the upper echelons of the bureaucracy and pay scale.

This enigmatic status syndrome persisted as a residual "psycho-social adversity" even after adjusting for naughty habits like smoking and excluding people who were overweight at the beginning of the time period, and showed no preference for more menial or lower-paid occupational categories. Chronic everyday stress appeared to be a biological mechanism, working directly on the neuro-endocrine and immune systems to reduce the body's resilience and, over time, upset its natural quest for homeostasis.[8]

Such findings, which are echoed in studies of migrant populations or forcibly resettled indigenous peoples, are remarkable. And yet the consensus is to glide past them, shrug, and point the finger at "Big Food."

That we opt to denounce our own food system may point to a broader unease about the world today. Supporting that is the striking result of the July 2015 Food Demand Survey, an innovative tool developed by Oklahoma State University's Jayson Lusk. Two-thirds of Americans said they would prefer to live in the past, and the number of the rest who would prefer to live more than 100 years into the future easily outstripped those expressing interest in the next 50 years.[9]

It may even be that the constant emphasis on the downside risks of food is throwing fuel on anxiety's fire. John Ioannidis, the iconoclastic director of the Stanford Prevention Research Center, grabbed a random set of recipes and picked out fifty typical ingredients – like lemons, onions, and bread – and found that the vast majority of them had been subject to a scientific study linking them to cancer, usually concluding that they posed an extra risk and drawing media attention.

Reading between the battle lines

Never waste a crisis, they say. The obesity-as-pandemic discourse has caught many industrial players on their heels. Food companies are bidding exorbitant sums to buy up smaller firms that have managed to generate a healthy allure. Drug companies, meanwhile, are keen to tap into a market that is literally bigger by the day.

One emblematic example of the relation between the obesity-as-pandemic discourse and industry is the career trajectory of Julie Gerberding. As director of the US Centers for Disease Control and Prevention, she described obesity as more serious than the "Black Death" which in the fourteenth century cut the global population by 25 percent. Criticized for having politicized health and climate change issues while there, she has moved on and was recently appointed executive vice president for strategic communications, global public policy and population health at Merck, one of the largest providers of the antibiotics used to speed up livestock growth. That practice has grown in step with Americans' body mass in another correlation of note.[10]

Insinuations of conflict of interest are a dime a dozen in the food policy arena today. In early 2015, the *British Medical Journal* ran a five-part investigative series decrying that public health scientists often take research funding and consultancy fees from companies being blamed for the obesity crisis. While naming Coca-Cola, Nestlé, GlaxoSmithKline, and Weight Watchers International, the series focused on sugar, saying its industry lobby regularly sought to obtain seats for its chosen "unbiased" experts on dietary guideline panels and in the food industry, noting that many firms have pledged to reduce the calories in their products but that only regulation will assure that this is reduced by even more. One installment criticized Mars, a global confectionery company, for voluntarily lowering its sugar count by reducing portion size, implying that wholesale product reformulation, rather than moderation, is the only acceptable path.[11]

The series, which named various prominent UK individuals, triggered high-profile newspaper headlines but also a slew of letters from prestigious nutritionists noting that while industry funding may pose risks, they are smaller than those posed by limited government research funds. Noting that research sponsorships are now routinely disclosed in published papers, Tom Sanders, an emeritus professor at King's College London who once reeled in a $5 million grant to his university from a company dealing in sugar and its substitutes, said claiming that industry grants ineluctably bend researchers offering public advice itself plays into the hands of a political agenda.[12]

The often vitriolic ways conflict-of-interest allegations are made in the world of nutritional discourse are fascinating and warrant academic studies on their own. As it happens, there has been such a study, and what it found is that bias is less present in scientific papers funded by industry than in those that are not!

Financial conflicts are a threat to science, but far from the only one, especially as academic futures can be determined by pressure to make a splash and the allocation of public money may also be influenced by the desire for what managerial culture now terms "actionable results." According to Dennis Bier, the editor-in-chief of the *American Journal of Clinical Nutrition*, "allegiance bias" is stronger than financial bias.[13] Such cases were empirically evident in the studies of "white hat bias" by Mark Cope and David Allison, who focused on the "distortion of information in the service of what may be perceived to be righteous ends."

They noted that research that supported breastfeeding, a WHO priority, was far more likely to be published in the first place than research that did not, or that even concluded with a null result – which is also one of the engines of science. They also noticed that the sole study the FDA cited as proving that new rules requiring listing nutritional information on restaurant menus help people make better decisions in fact showed that was only true, and very modestly, for the choices parents made for their children.

The authors then turned specifically to obesity. They looked at two prominent studies on the consumption of sweetened beverages – one of them titled "Preventing Childhood Obesity" – and found a spin ratio of two to one in the way that research was eventually cited and used.

The primary finding of the studies, both of which were based on experiments comparing how adolescents respond to consuming sodas or being kept from drinking them, was that no change in BMI took place even over periods of a year. A minor finding was that BMI did rise for soda drinkers who were already substantially overweight or obese. Analysis of the citations of those papers found that research done without industry funding had a strong tendency to trumpet the second point and ignore the first one.[14]

Cope and Allison blame press releases for misrepresenting the data and journalists for parroting clichés that contribute to the general sanctimony. Engaging in hyperbole of their own to conclude, they draw a comparison to the way wartime propagandists "dehumanize the enemy to inflame spirits" and facilitate massacres!

Another important strategy in making claims about obesity has to do with releasing more public money. After all, the purpose of the story about predicting the date of 100 percent obesity was – as indicated in its own title – to make a claim about the likely cost of such a fate. That was described as destined to rise to almost $1 trillion a year by 2030 in the US alone. That's five times the current cost, including that due to productivity losses, according to a study conducted by the Society of Actuaries on commission for the insurance industry, which invented the BMI index and has money on the table.[15] Such forecasts are made for planning purposes; insurers project the value of claims for underwriting purposes, while others float a higher figure in hopes of setting a benchmark for savings that will entice the government to open its purse strings.

A crystal-clear variant of the logic came in 2015 when the WHO released a study on air pollution, saying it causes one in four Europeans to die prematurely and imposes economic costs or almost $2 trillion a year or 10 percent of GDP – more than the total personal income tax burden on the continent![16] Alluding to dividends that might flow from reducing pollution, WHO's regional director for Europe, Zsuzsanna Jakab, said the study "provides decision-makers across the whole of government with a compelling reason to act."

That does sound like a fully-fledged emergency. How should the money, if it is ever authorized, be spent? In the obesity space, food and beverage companies trumpet the idea that fat can be exercised away, so sponsor fitness programs and urge the state to provide more playgrounds, an enticingly cheaper solution albeit one involving direct upfront costs and tough urban planning choices. The trillion-dollar claim, meanwhile, comes from the medical community.

Pharmaceutical companies are keen on having obesity classified as a disease so that the doors of insurance companies may be thrown open for their curative therapies. They are making progress. In 2013, the American Medical Association approved that classification after a lopsided floor vote defied the advice of a committee the doctors' own lobby had set up to study the question. And in the summer of 2015, a bipartisan legislative bill called the "Treat and Reduce Obesity Act" was introduced to a congressional committee. If passed it will oblige Medicare to include weight-loss treatments on the list of reimbursable services, at least for senior citizens.[17] The Obesity Action Council, a non-profit organization whose three "platinum" funders are Takeda, Novo Nordisk, and Eisai, three foreign multinationals that have released new anti-obesity drugs in the past eighteen months, hailed the bill being floored.

Surprisingly, given the magnitude of the potential client base and the antiquity of the ailment, there is no category-killing weight-loss drug. Some anti-obesity pills were pulled due to adverse side effects, while a trickle of newer ones appear to have had only a modest impact. Some doctors offer bariatric surgery, where the size of a patient's stomach is reduced and food is re-routed away from the intestine. Once considered an invasive and risky operation for use only when a person's BMI is above 40, its popularity is growing. Indeed, the *Journal of the American Medical Association* reported in the summer of 2015 that it is a more effective means to weight loss than any other and touted the idea that it should be used earlier and more often.[18]

The pharmaceutical industry has an explanation for why it doesn't have a viable anti-obesity drug but could develop one: investment is low due to "a challenging regulatory and reimbursement environment and associated commercial uncertainty."

More than a quarter of US health care costs are linked to obesity, but only 0.2 percent of related spending goes on bariatric surgery and a negligible 0.04 percent of total drug expenditure goes on anti-obesity therapies, according to Pierre-Yves Cremieux, a managing principal at Boston-based consultancy Analysis Group and the author of the above phrase. He is bullish on the fact that four new drugs have been approved after a decade-long drought, noting that they basically operate as appetite suppressants and promise to achieve the "clinically meaningful" effect of triggering weight loss of 5 percent.[19] That level is deemed a big success by Weight Watchers, a popular points-based dietary program. Patients often expect more, so often drop out of voluntary drug-based weight-loss schemes.

But assured insurance reimbursement, through national health programs or private providers, would boost long-term use of current anti-obesity drugs, says Katharine Andino, in charge of obesity marketing in the USA for Takeda Pharmaceuticals. Global revenue for such products has dwindled to only $359 million, an unviable figure for an industry that spends more than that just to develop a new drug.[20] Meanwhile, shortly after Cremieux reported on the woes of obesity, his colleagues released another report on the scourge of depression, calculating that it imposed a $210 billion burden on the US economy – that's roughly the same as diabetes and close to half as much as obesity in general.[21]

Spin is inevitable, abundant and more or less follows predictable patterns. For example, early in 2015 the *Pharmaceutical Journal* ran a headline reporting "Finnish study explores association between statin use and diabetes" and alluding to "slightly" increased risks of Type 2 diabetes for the millions of people taking cholesterol-lowering statins after being advised they were at risk of a stroke. The study reviewed 8,749 people aged 45 to 73 for six years and found that those taking statins – a hefty quarter of the sample – were 46 percent more likely to have developed diabetes over the period than those who did not.[22] That's tantamount to drinking a six-pack of cola a day.

While activists naturally enjoy hyperbole, excess distorting of the facts seriously drains credibility from the policy debate. Add the estimated tabs for pollution, depression, and obesity to historic state functions such as education, building roads and bridges, defense, ordinary health care, and providing for survival in old age starts to seem like a hopeless task, as taxpayers may take their chances rather than vote to go to flea markets for clothes and buy the cheapest calories available.

One example of such hyperbolic discounting comes in a breezy essay on the epidemiology of obesity by Philip James, the founder of World Obesity and the main voice behind calls for an absolute cap on free sugars intake at 5 percent of calories and now a new plea to push it below 3 percent. That is tantamount to an 80 percent sugar reduction in countries such as the UK, USA, Germany, and South Africa.[23]

Noting how extra weight creeps up on the body and then demands to be maintained with yet higher food consumption, Dr. James blames "marketing experts" for unleashing a wave of highly energy-dense easy-to-eat foods. These have muscled fresh products off supermarket shelves and created a habit of "grazing" that make proper meals ever less frequent and besets the brain with constant temptation, leaving consumers powerlessly in their thrall. The solution, he raffishly insists, will require not just heavy-handed regulation of retail products but a revamping of agriculture so that fruits and vegetables can regain their pride of place.[24] It's a thrilling vision. Fortunately, reversing the effects of fifty years of postwar agricultural subsidies should be a "relatively small" affair and no big deal for farmers, he claims in closing, citing a study that found that the USA would have to add only 2 percent of arable land to its current cropland.

But the US Department of Agriculture study from 1999 he cited didn't say that at all. It proposed to model what would have to happen to American farmland in order to bring it more in line with the government's dietary recommendation. It did in fact calculate the need for a net increase of 5.6 million acres, so there's the 2 percent, but the entire point of the exercise was to look at the required shifts in cultivation. Most of the sugar cane and sugar beet fields would have to go, but they are tiny. It was the tripling of the land put to citrus fruits, the doubling of that for melons and berries, and the quadrupling of the acreage devoted to dark green, leafy vegetables that appeared to defy details like seasons, climate and the rules of nature.[25]

The authors, government economists Edwin Young and Linda Scott Kantor, said the adjustment would be sharp and "complicated" by the small detail that many crops are persnickety about soils and can't just be grown anywhere. Such a shift to fresh produce would entail what they delicately termed "significant price adjustments" across the board and still require the kind of foreign policy that can guarantee a hefty flow of imports.

In the end, such a shift would be a historical drama and neither the environment nor food safety would enjoy it; ironically, increased food processing would emerge as the sole mitigating option. Many may champion such a shift nonetheless, and they may be wise, but it would be an epic affair.

That's even more evident in the wake of reports that many of the greenest eaters in the world, living in Marin County near San Francisco, are suffering from chronic fatigue, hair loss, and more as the result of inadvertently consuming a lethal poison mentioned in an Agatha Christie novel and used tactically to knock off unwanted spouses and political opponents. Thallium accumulates in soils near where coal was burned or cement made, and is happily taken up by cruciferous vegetables including broccoli, collard greens and, in particular, kale, the booming superfood that is all the rage in California for healthy salads and juices. In fact, scientists recommend kale as a tool to clean up contaminated sites, as it pulls copious amounts of thallium into its leaves.[26]

Those keen on eluding the clutches of the epidemic-manufacturing Big Food vendors of cheap hyper-processed obesity pellets should also keep an extra eye out for *Campylobacter jejuni*, one of the world's most persistent bacterial torments. Marc Bellemare, an economics professor at the University of Minnesota, found after two years of gathering and crunching data that outbreaks and cases of the dreaded bug and related food-borne illness vectors increased in step with the number of farmers' markets, which have quintupled in number in the USA since the mid-1990s. Fortunately that's just a correlation.[27]

Human ingenuity can no doubt overcome these drawbacks, but even the modest amount of extra land needed would require razing the last fifteen years' worth of residential and business construction in the country, according to the 2012 census. To be sure, such sweeping evictions and dismantling of enterprises would likely be worth avoiding a repeat of the bubonic plague, but one does hope that policy-makers engaging on such a path are extremely sure that's what they are preventing and have an equitable plan to smooth out the inconveniences. And as more than half the increased average weight of Americans occurred among people born before 1939, since which time they have become taller, blaming current subsidies for grains and sugar will still leave quite a lot of work to do.[28]

And as it happens, it's not just the USA that is short of fruit and vegetables. Globally, three-fourths of the world population eats less than the WHO's recommended 600 grams or five servings a day, and if everyone started to comply with that target, the world would face a 22 percent production shortfall, with that figure rising to well above 85 percent in many African countries. Crunching FAO data and factoring in the fact that fresh produce tends to spoil quickly, the global supply of fruit and vegetables is only two-thirds of what is needed.[29]

Such nice little mice

Most of the reports we read about how sugar causes not just obesity but addiction, emotional moods, cretinism and more, begin their journey with mice. Laboratory mice are routinely fed "western" diets – mostly potato chips, in one case – to see how their bodies react. This is an established practice, to which has been added the genetic splicing and dicing of the animals to single out factors for focused investigation. While sometimes other animals are used – Chinese scientists are playing up the silk worm as a human metabolic model – mice are particularly excellent because our genomes are quite similar and because they grow and breed so fast.[30, 31]

Early researchers, in their effort to create obese rats for testing, found that the best way was to feed them fats. In fact, diets with 66 percent sucrose were dubbed the "best" healthy diet, a low-fat menu designed as a control in hopes that a high-fat diet consisting mostly of Crisco, at the time crystallized cottonseed oil, would spur the rats to bigger weight gains. That's just what it did in a 1955 experiment done by US government scientists in Washington, as the Crisco rats reached a kilogram at 41 weeks of age, almost twice the weight of their sucrose-slurping peers.[32]

Times change. An experiment almost sixty years later fed obese rats a high-fat ad libitum diet to see what would happen if they were allowed to eat as much as they wanted but for only eight hours a day as opposed to having night-time access to the trough. It was found that rats in a relative rush ate as many calories but had normal glucose tolerance, improved motor function, and less adiposity, all of which were attributed to their respect of the natural circadian clock governing when to sleep.[33]

That maps the human experience. It has been noted in several children's studies as well as by the Nurses' Health Study, one of the longest-running cohort studies in the world and conducted on 60,000 medical professionals in the USA, that those who slept least had a 30 percent higher likelihood of gaining 30 pounds within two decades and a 15 percent higher chance of becoming obese. With fragmented shift work increasingly common in the modern workforce, a third of Americans now getting less than six hours of sleep a night, and with medical errors accounting for a multiple of obesity-related deaths and often attributed to exhaustion, there might be merit in policy support for what the analysts call "sleep hygiene."[34]

Just as sleep is an issue for both mice and men, we also share a predilection for especially palatable foods.

It has been shown that rats that dine on a so-called cafeteria diet – including goodies like cakes, cookies, Froot Loops, cereals and savory snacks – will if freely allowed take up twice as much energy as their peers eating only standard chow, and that they shift away from mealtimes to a constant snacking regime. And whereas rats tired from running in their wheel have an unerring eye for carbohydrates – the fastest-acting energy source – well-fed rats like gooier stuff.[35]

There are countless experiments, but one of the more interesting ones found that it's not really sugar nor fat but the combination that is doing us in. Offering rats three menus – high-fat high-sugar, high-fat, or high-sugar – all alongside access to standard chow – the researchers were keen to track body weight gain as well as plasma leptin concentrations and examine how a key hypothalamic peptide involved in governing our appetite reacted. Left to their own devices, rodents usually overeat high-fat or high-energy foods initially but then compensate by lowering their calorie intake. The question, then, is what might make them stop compensating. It turned out that rats eating the high-sugar diet did not change any of the key blood indicators, nor did they put on weight compared to rats eating just chow. The high-fat rats also didn't put on any extra weight. But the third group, eating the high fat high-sugar diet, did. It's the combination that may drive hyperphagia – overeating – and eventual obesity, the scientists conclude.[36]

The logical conclusion from this and the thousands of other experiments done, usually with an eye to identify a smoking gun, is that our food woes reflect our whole diet and not a single thing. You can have that criminal cinnamon roll but don't offset it later with milk chocolate. Although advocating a balanced diet is nothing new, the idea that certain combinations of food have synergies that can be detrimental – or positive in some cases – is intriguing.

It is known that food preparation techniques can have a significant impact on the way dietary energy balances work, which is presumably relevant for those who formulate guidelines. For example, Burmese pythons fed ground or cooked meat used 13 percent less energy to digest it. Grinding and cooking meat led to savings nearly twice as large, suggesting that, all else being exactly equal, those who enjoy a pricey steak tartare are less likely to get fat than those having a burger. Snakes, of course, sleep it off, but humans may not.[37]

Something to process

The role of combination lies behind ancient culinary traditions, most of which used spices and herbs not just for taste and to mitigate spoilage but also to generate additional nutritional benefits. Capsaicin, the hot element in chili peppers, raises energy expenditure, so pile it on. Oregano, meanwhile, inhibits absorption of iron.[38] Sugar may lack micronutrients but affects the way others are taken and in fact increases the bioavailability of non-heme iron, a point of relevance given that iron deficiency is a serious health problem for an estimated 1.6 billion people worldwide.[39]

Scientists in Ohio recently decided to test how curcumin, the phytochemical heart of turmeric and an active mitigator of inflammation in the human digestive system, worked on mice. The problem was the animals pooped most of it out. Their Midwestern human subjects also pushed it right through, absorbing almost none of its beneficial effects. As it happens, research in the land of curry has already shown that turmeric actually goes into action when accompanied by black pepper. The Ohio solution was to feed the rodents a nano-emulsion variant they have developed which would also work for people who don't like spicy Indian food.[40]

As expected, ingesting the curcumin helped lower the endotoxin count – or lipopolysaccharides, usually written as LPS and a common stage-setter for both obesity and diabetes – of the rats, indicating that turmeric can help fight obesity and diabetes. Remarkably, it also worked best on laboratory rather than wild-type rats, suggesting it might be doubly effective on those eating the western diet.[41]

Such discoveries are particularly relevant in the public discourses on obesity and sugar. Herbs and spices are nutritional wizards with insignificant calorie loads that need accompaniment, a point the processed foods industry might take to heart. Sugar is well-placed to serve as the provider of palatability to help people eat more of these metabolically beneficial foods. Given existing food supplies and tastes, such a fortification approach would be a far more affordable and less drastic route to public health than many of the others being floated.

While some worry that food fortification would just be a gift to industry, it is part of the established toolkit and is more efficacious than supplements. Few mention that the primary customers of the $40 billion US vitamin supplement industry today are in fact already the healthiest Americans, boasting a range of traits from higher income and physical activity to lower BMIs. As things are, American youth get more than half of their vitamin D, thiamine, and folate from fortified foods, as well as a third of their vitamin A, C, B-6, B-12, riboflavin, niacin, and iron, while those at the greatest risk of poverty, obesity, and poor health are those who use supplements the least.[42]

The role of economic class is hardly part of any American exceptionalism. Consider Brazil, where obesity is widespread and which actually has a higher mortality rate for non-communicable diseases than the USA or UK. Consumption of biscuits and bread has risen 21 percent over a decade and a half, suggesting that highly-processed foods may be the culprit, even though local sugar intake has always been high. Given what is known about the role of dietary fibers in impeding intestinal inflammation, the 20 percent drop in consumption of green vegetables and fruit may be the core problem.[43]

A closer look indicates that the latter foods are expensive, the former cheap, and that obesity among higher socioeconomic status women has been declining since 1989. Back then, a third of the country was hungry. The solution surely must not lie in reducing calories but in finding a way to add nutritional elements where they are missing. Fresh foods are surely the best, but demanding that lower-income people spend more money on healthier food – whose availability has actually decreased during Brazil's economic boom – will not be sustainable. Unless working-class incomes start rising faster than others, which has not happened anywhere for decades, spurning workarounds doesn't seem prudent.

Brazilians now take 52 percent of their energy calories from foods rich in solid fats and added sugars, which compares to British or Canadian levels and reflects a virtual infrastructure of distribution and habit that may prove hard to change. However, saying that food companies won't do it because it will reduce their profit makes no sense unless to imply somewhat preposterously that policies are free and prices need not rise.[44]

A practical approach of recognizing food processing techniques for their role in food safety and preservation along with their potential to increase delivery of nutrients in a bio-available form comes from India, a country with serious hunger and malnutrition issues as well as the painful history of beriberi, a disease caused by new rice-milling techniques introduced in the late nineteenth century that took decades to understand. Microbiologists there note that processing allows for fortification to tackle malnutrition, and as a dynamic industry ought to be applied to more traditional indigenous foods known for their flavonoid and antioxidant values to supplement dietary nutrient shortfalls further.[45]

On a more banal level, it's also possible – researchers have shown this, too![46] – that one way to get recalcitrant pre-schoolers to eat broccoli is to offer it to them with a sweet-and-fat-tinged dip. That's not so ridiculous; most people burn out on the sweet taste over time but not everyone develops a liking for bitter tastes.

A psychological turn

As noted, the curcumin benefited the laboratory rats more than the wild-type ones. That highlights the fact that rodents are having an obesity pandemic of their own. Use of lab mice began on a mass scale in the postwar era and became even more advanced when scientists learned how to "knock out" various chromosomes to allow researchers to focus singly on specific traits and reactions.

The rodents themselves tend to live protected from predators in cages and, while incredibly bored, most enjoy an ad libitum diet, meaning they can eat all of the chow pellets they want. Those subject to restricted diets can live for more than four years, whereas those on ad libitum diets never seem to make it past two and a half years. The reason is that their hormones, glucose, insulin, leptin, cholesterol, and triglyceride levels are out of whack. In short, the caged and now dim-witted creatures tend to avoid the exercise wheel, carry around as much as half their body weight in fat, and are always already metabolically morbid. This is before they start their career as research subjects for drug tests.

In fact, the insulin sensitivity of mice that are shifted to a meal plan, which translates into a cut in calorie intake of at least 20 percent, increases by half. The message for humans is clear: One fairly surefire way to lose weight and improve various metabolic markers is to eat less in general.

Some say, only half in jest, that the fat mice may be the perfect model for *Homo sapiens* as we now are. That could be: some medical drug therapies that worked on mice in trials have only worked on obese people, and when then tested on specially-raised lean mice, they also didn't work.

One source of confusion in nutrition research is that obesity and associated ailments can make ordinary functions go into reverse. That may explain a recent finding that a diet of fiber-rich rye bread did not, as expected, change the demographics of gut bacteria of a group of adults with metabolic syndrome in Finland. While it is refreshing to see a published study reporting a null result, the experiment may not mean that dietary fibers are not critical contributors to metabolic health but merely that – as with the rats – the mechanics change when disease is already present. Therapy, in short, is different from health maintenance, just as people with diabetes cutting back on sugar doesn't at all mean that sugar caused their condition.

Revelation of the laboratory rat's sorry state comes thanks to a seminal contribution from Bronwen Martin, a US government scientist, who reckons that hundreds of initially promising cancer therapies and some for Alzheimer's disease have failed because they didn't work except in conditions resembling the laboratory. Testing her hypothesis by subjecting rats to different feeding rhythms – calorie restriction and alternate-day fasting – she found that animals reacted not only with different maze-solving skills and cholesterol levels but even by forming different genes for various bodily tissues.[47]

That, to be sure, suggests that constant consumption of little more than sucrose, potato chips, and cookies, with an occasional pepperoni pizza on the side, does over time lead epigenetically at the very least to obesity. So don't make that your diet!

If the fact that laboratory rodents have become so peculiar weakens their utility as models for the remaining "wild-type" humans, the same may be true for the increasing number of studies focusing on how sugar's real demonic attributes are neurological in nature.[48] Another spicy report from the laboratory suggested that sugar overconsumption triggers a chronic depression in the way our brains process incentives that takes place specifically in adolescence and may cause problems of a mostly psychiatric nature later. In this case, rats were given a hefty bolt of sucrose early on, and then showed "decreased motivation" for sweet-tasting things as adults. The authors reckon essentially that the overexposure ended up numbing the reward system. And while they note that reduced neurologically-driven desire for junk food might be just what the doctor ordered regarding obesity, they worry that such lack of motivation could be a precursor to depression or drug addiction.[49]

Apparently, then, since adolescents are by far the age cohort for whom sugar intake is the largest – added-sugar intake by adolescents is about 50 percent higher than the national average for adults in the USA and Brazil and accounts for more than 17 percent of all calories consumed by American youth – we have an escape route: instead of all being overweight by 2048, we can all just get high. That might be a regulatory battle far more intense than any today!

Call it the psychological turn. Much of the new work on sugar now being done on humans is in fact about behavioral reward systems that quickly slip into moralistic clichés. Several scholars have suggested that sweets and junk food are intrinsically desirable and that the only way people can avoid eating them is through masterful displays of self-control. For example, a new Canadian study used theta burst stimulation on young women volunteers, pumping transcranial magnetic pulses to a functional part of the brain associated with planning ahead and abstract reasoning. They responded to the treatment, which is increasingly used in cases of major depression, by gulping down 70 grams more of junk food than the controls who were given a sham theta burst. The authors conclude that sugar and other high-calorie foods are indeed a primordial craving and will take control of people unable to exercise what they call strong "executive functions."

In a similar vein, a California research team concluded that stress triggers neural pathways that stoke desire for palatable comfort foods and push some people towards eating habits that over time can increase the risk of obesity. Translated, that means that if you are persistently down and out you may perhaps seek out some cheap liquor – as Hogarth documented a few centuries ago.

Some of the experiments being done imply that policy-makers might have to give some clearer instruction to Hollywood on what constitutes a healthy plot. People who watched a sad movie ate 28 percent more popcorn than peers who watched a light comedy in a test setting, and apparently even more in the wild, according to the amount of leftover popcorn thrown in the trash at some cinema malls. So now you know: poignant drama is obesogenic.[50]

One useful takeaway from the newer tests is that they increasingly test for and mention stress, which is considered a serious cause of endocrinological and cardiovascular woes.

The US Department of Defense long ago funded research that found that repeated chronic stress leads to weight loss even when rats' leptin levels – which trigger hunger signals – are artificially boosted. Of course, combat duty – the human parallel – does not last forever, and acute stress is not the same as the chronic kind.

It may be that fat rats know what, within their limited options, they are doing. Researchers in Beirut fed a high-carbohydrate chow diet with extra chocolate cookies and peanut butter to rats in prettified cages and subjected them to daily stress tests. The rats put on weight but managed to lower their levels of corticosterone, a key stressing steroid that when in constant oversupply appears to trigger diabetic syndromes. For them, comfort food was a boon.

Meanwhile, in Australia, a similar trial was set up, except in this case the rats were given a surprise change in diet to see how they reacted. The cookie-eaters, who had become chubbier, became upset and started eating notably less while posting higher levels of the genetic programming molecule associated with stress, major depression, and hypoglycemia. The other set happily began eating cookies and enjoying reduced levels of fear-and-anxiety in the amygdala, part of the brain's reward system. "These findings have implications for dieting in humans," the authors note.[51]

So it seems the battle of the bulge leaves us facing some stark choices. We can all become peasants in an overhauled global agricultural system, we can start taking drugs, or we can accept chronic stress, which will lead us to obesity or addiction anyway. That makes me want to eat 28 percent more popcorn already.

While chatting on the sidelines of an event about food at the Milan Expo, Robert Gibson – a prolific nutrition scholar and now professor of functional food science at the University of Adelaide in Australia – told me not to panic. "I've been working in nutrition for forty years, during which I've learned many things, and almost all of them were wrong," he said. "Weight is over-rated." He said he liked the standard advice that people should eat food, not too much of it, and remember their dietary fibers. "But 'don't worry' should be tacked on any food rules," he added.

Dubito Ergo Sum

4

All things are poison and nothing is without poison; only the dose makes a thing not a poison.

Philippus Aureolus Theophrastus Bombastus von Hohenheim, aka Paracelsus

A review of the nutritional analyses and scientific work on sugar shows that by and large its relation to adverse health dynamics is based on correlations, some striking, some less so, and one is left somehow unconvinced that sugar on its own is a toxic demon.

There are many people, many cultures, and many diets. While obesity and corollary problems have cropped up with an alarming global regularity, there are many potential non-food causes for that, and the most solid nutritional rule of thumb with universal applicability seems not to be to cut out any single element but to redouble efforts not to forget dietary fibers, ideally with colorful leaves, on the grounds that they carry and provide many of the inputs we need for enzymatic processes we've partly outsourced to our gut biota. It's their lack that is almost always the gaping hole in our alimentary health.

But there are two strands related to sugar that have left this author perplexed. One has to do with HFCS (high-fructose corn syrup), the well-known name for an ingredient widely used in sweetened beverages but also often in a slew of branded food products including breakfast cereals, candies, crackers, cough syrups, pancake mixes, salad dressings and barbecue sauces, ketchups and soups, even pickles and many types of whole-grain bread. The other has to do with something with a very technical and rarely-heard name, Advanced Glycation Endproducts (AGEs), found in processed foods but also made by our body and ultimately the product of fire. So this intermezzo chapter will try to explain the state of knowledge.

The F-word

Fructose and glucose together make up almost all of what we mean by "refined sugar." Considered on its own, fructose is notably soluble and has a faster-acting impact on taste than its partner. Perhaps for that reason it is suspected of packing an especially powerful punch that even makes us forget we consumed it. Fructose does not generate an insulin response and as its glycemic index is very low, it could be a management hassle for people who are already diabetic and monitor that index.

According to Dr. Lustig, while almost all life forms know how to use and usually even need glucose, fructose is not an essential part of metabolism and thus overworks the liver, triggering abundant triglycerides which signal higher risks for cardiovascular disease. As it does not trigger satiety signals, this could allow overconsumption, although whether it actively does so by fiddling with our neurological reward systems has not been established. It is, as the headline-friendly title of one of his latest paper says, "alcohol without the buzz."[1]

It also features loudly in the name of the cornstarch-derived HFCS introduced in the US in the 1970s and now widely used, especially in the beverage industry. As many focus on the link between increased caloric intake and the substantial increase in consumption of sweetened beverages in recent decades – they now contribute four times more calories than they did in the 1960s – it is natural to wonder about whether this new entry to the food supply is a harbinger of woe.[2]

For the most part, it is sugary beverages in general rather than HFCS that is sparking nutritionists' ire. A high-profile study announced in the summer of 2015 that such drinks cause 184,000 deaths a year, more than two-thirds of which are due to diabetes. Mexico, the world's leading consumer of such beverages by far, led the tables with 405 deaths for every 1 million, with the USA coming second at a rate of around a third of that. Once again the claim, actually a repeat of statistical research done two years earlier that had failed to elicit public interest, was based on crunching gobs of data on mortality and commercial availability, and one of the lead authors has openly said he favors eradicating sugary beverages from the food supply.

The study showed two of the stylistic quirks common to such epidemiological studies: first, it was written up in a way that contextually describes the alleged causal role of the selected villain in health woes as a given, and, second, it emphasized the potential efficacy of appearing to combat a major scourge by eliminating a "single, modifiable component of diet." Just as predictable was the response by the American beverage industry, which urged people to get exercise, oddly linked diabetes risk to ethnic minorities, and added a historical anecdote about atherosclerosis cases in ancient Egypt.[3]

The arrival of HFCS and the ensuing boom of sodas has triggered substantial investigation, in one case leading Dutch researchers to commission a special orange-colored soda using almost only fructose to try out on university students. HFCS is not widely used in Europe, where C4 plants like corn are not prevalent. HFCS in fact consists of both glucose and fructose, with the latter accounting for 42 percent for standard formulas used with liquids and 55 percent for those in dry foods. However, actual percentages can vary quite sharply, suggesting that some of its use in manufacturing processes is not homogeneous.[4]

As already noted, abundant claims can be made, and methodologies can be wobbly. Some of the tests using mice involve feeding them fructose calories which for humans would translate into roughly four 44-ounce super big gulps of soda a day. While adverse outcomes at that level warrant theoretical study, there are very few people capable of knocking back what amounts to more than two six-packs each and every day. Using one published claim that one extra serving of a soft drink per day would lead to 50 kilograms or 110 pounds of extra weight after ten years, such consumption would presumably lead to people weighing more than half a ton![5]

One classic study published in the journal produced by Dr. James's organization in 2009 claimed to be "the first study to show that excessive intake of fructose can cause almost all of the features of metabolic syndrome." Written by two researchers with patent applications for obesity-related treatments, it found that a quarter of overweight adults on the Spanish island of Mallorca developed new-onset metabolic syndrome after drinking 200 grams of liquid fructose a day for two weeks on top of their ordinary eating habits, which included around 55 grams already.

These already overweight volunteers sipped slowly throughout the day, eating 175 calories less in ordinary foods and still took in an extra 600 calories a day. One in nine of those tested dropped out due to intense diarrhea caused by an amount of fructose equal to roughly eight times the recommended amount and twice the amount of total sugars even the most energy-starved American adolescents manage if they try. Don't try that experiment at home![6]

The Dutch study that made the special HFCS carbonated soda to test in Europe plied the drinks in high but plausible doses on people ahead of meal times and found there were no differences in energy intake or satiety effects, between drinking beverages containing HFCS, ordinary sucrose, or in fact milk. That finding has been repeated, with no postprandial differences in blood glucose, insulin or other concentrations found between beverages containing HFCS and sucrose, which in any case presumably breaks into its monosaccharide components in the highly acidic environment of a soft drink.[7]

Such studies proliferated after HFCS came into the spotlight in the wake of published correlations between the product's introduction to the food system and increasing obesity rates. One of the authors of that correlation later told *The New York Times* that their paper was "a theory meant to spur science, but it's quite possible that it may be found out not to be true."[8]

That author, Barry Popkin, is a professor at the University of North Carolina with a prolific publishing trajectory and a career clearly dedicated to the nutritional problems of the world's poorest, which began while he was an undergraduate from Wisconsin living in a Delhi slum.

His is stellar and fascinating globe-trotting work. In fact, his interests are so wide that he and his research colleagues have produced copious studies attributing the obesity epidemic to dietary fats, to sugar in general, to HFCS, to soft drinks, to fast foods, to snacks, and even to portion sizes. The common trend there – apart from ready-made media impacts – is the assumption that obesity is driven by the fact that too many people eat too much. That is almost certainly true but perhaps cannot serve as much of a pretext for singling out a single dietary element. Indeed, almost all the scientists who consider sugar a food rather than a poison still say that it is a great element to cut back on in any weight-loss agenda due to its lack of any nutrient baggage.

Even Popkin is moving on. In a later paper on HFCS, catchily titled "is this what's for dinner?" he noted that HFCS consumption trends were trailing off and might do so sharply if Washington revamped agricultural subsidies that benefit corn growers. He warned nutritionists of overlooking other types of added caloric sweeteners – which is pertinent, because one risk of stigmatizing or merely capping a given product is that legions lie in the wings to take its place.[9]

Fructose in extreme cases could probably turn our liver into foie gras, Luc Tappy, one of the foremost experts on the subject, told me. "Look, it's quite likely that sugar contributes to increased body weight, but it's not specific to sugar, it's about overconsumption," he said.

Fructose itself may even be a godsend at times, offering tactical advantages to athletes, according to Tappy, whose laboratory in Switzerland does a lot of detective work on fructose. Physical exercise needs a continuous supply of energy to the working muscle, whose efforts at the same time sharply increases glucose oxidation, leading to muscle fatigue. Given that challenge, fructose can offer a helping hand because when it is metabolized it helps produce glucose. Sports-drinks makers are probably right in experimenting to find the right level of fructose to add to their potions, he says, but these are strictly for situations of peak physical activity and not jogging in the park.[10]

Pure fructose can help elite athletes avoid hitting the wall, as happens to more than 40 percent of runners in competitive marathons as they run out of energy and struggle to keep pace due to the fact their muscles are oxidizing carbohydrates faster than any new source can offset.[11]

The reason fructose might be useful in such situations – which entail acute rather than chronic stress – is precisely because it is a fast-acting compound. The natural fructose in fruit, by contrast, is dispersed through the fibers of a complex food, which likely means it doesn't leap into action all at once. That explains why many people prefer a candy bar instead of fruit before a big game; they want their energy pronto.

Curiously, research based on the kind of direct human dietary intervention deemed impossible today was once done. Almost fifty years ago, doctors in South Africa obliged seventeen Bantu and white adults to eat twenty servings of fruit a day, along with nuts and avocados to provide fat. That translates to around 200 grams of fructose, so in line with the Mallorca experiment in quantity, but taken in the form of fruit fibers instead of a distilled liquid in a special bottle. After three to six months, there were no adverse effects; insulin levels rose sharply in some cases at the beginning but then settled back to normal.[12] While few people can manage eating so much fruit – the subjects were volunteers, but may have had incentives – the reason for the untroubled and even beneficial nature of the reaction in this case likely lies in the fact that sugar in fruit takes longer to break down and so there is no energy rush. Maybe that's why there's so much faddish talk about chewing more, and more slowly. There'll soon be an app for that.[13]

So fructose may tick the f-for-fake box in natural terms. The same might be said of wine, of course, and that was precisely what Dr. Lustig was getting at.

Endgame

Advanced glycation endproducts, henceforth AGEs in line with their standard acronym, are the derivatives of interactions between glucose and protein or glucose and lipids. They are a wildly diverse gang of highly oxidant compounds that have been strongly linked to diabetes and may also be a driver of obesity and even physical lassitude or exhaustion. Despite the thousands of clinical, laboratory, epidemiological, sociological, and psychological research programs devoted to sugar, remarkably little is known about AGEs or what they do.

The first thing to note is that they are the product of a combination, in which a simple sugar – glucose, which our brain relies on for fuel – binds to an amino acid in a process driven by heat and conducted without the help of any enzyme. It's essentially a chemical rather than a biological event, and, with no offense to raw foods, it is behind some truly memorable culinary moments.

When our Paleolithic ancestors sat around the campfire and invented culture while grilling their meat, an act that maximized their energy extraction from the meal and allowed them to spend less than a fifth of the time eating as our primate cousins, they were packing in AGEs. AGEs form by what is now called the Maillard reaction, named after a French chemist who discovered it a century ago, although it would be another fifty years before it was studied in more detail by those who prepare food for others. Chefs, in particular, are big fans of the Maillard reaction, as deploying it is a crafty skill that bestows unique favors. Think caramelized onion, or basically any cooking effect that results in food browning and the emergence of pleasant scents and flavors.

Making has prevailed over knowing AGEs, as they have been engineered countless times but their description remains enigmatic. Cooking has many purposes, including making some foods more palatable and, as the beef-eating python demonstrated, more readily convertible into energy. It is also an established way to whack pathogens before they whack you. This is true in reverse; eating only raw foods is a fairly surefire way to lose weight, and those for whom it is a dietary regime tend to eat as much as they like and often still feel constantly hungry. An estimated 50 percent of the energy value of resistant starches and residual glucose in raw foods tends to elude the person who eats them so they end up fermented by intestinal microbes who convert some of them into short fatty acids.[14]

Cooking meat will gradually toughen the muscle fibers of flesh, but will also gelatinize the collagen sprinkled among those fibers, with the result being that it is easier to chew. That offers the desired succulence that, for example, traditional sun-dried beef jerky does not have.

The higher temperature of cooking triggers the Maillard reaction, which in turn produces a flavor that primates who never discovered fire cannot make but do seem to like. The ensuing AGEs, however, will ultimately take some of the protein deep into the colon where it will be hacked by microbes who then release detrimental compounds into our body, which may end up lodging in fat tissue or even the bloodstream and impede normal metabolic processes.

So there is a trade-off: humans eat tastier food and have more time for cultural pursuits, but at the cost of shaking up traditional digestion and having more uric acid slosh around. Today, of course, we have added agriculture to the repertoire and so no longer strictly need to eat meat.

The downside was likely quite limited in the early days. Taking a group of bushmen in Southern Africa as a proxy for the Paleolithic, one anthropologist noted that campfires extended the day and allowed a new form of social interaction. While daytime chitchat among the Ju/'hoan people tends to be about business plans and dividend policies, mostly about foraging and arguments over distribution, that's all turned off in the evening, which is a time for stories, singing and dancing.[15]

Evidently people had mastered the Maillard reaction long before it was discovered by science – or perhaps by the military, since so much of food processing was driven by the desire to keep soldiers' morale up. It is crucial not just to the aroma of Cheez-Whiz but also to those of roasted coffee or barbecued meats and is why bakeries smell the way they do. John Hodge, an African-American chemist in Peoria, Illinois, was the first to figure out its mechanics, which he shared in a 1953 paper that went on to become one of the all-time most cited pieces of scientific work.

A sugar and an amino acid bind, shedding some water and an unstable element that then undergoes what are known as "Amadori rearrangements" which produce a slew of compounds that in turn produce special traits ranging from color and smell to flavor and texture. The sheer number of reactions is one reason why so little is known about their exact role in the food system. Chefs and food manufacturers have figured out how to obtain effects but the cause remains elusive.

Some of the effects are unwelcome, such as the Maillard reactions that lead to acrylamide, a carcinogen, in French fries. It's present in a tiny amount, but then some people eat a lot of fries. Interestingly, the discovery of acrylamide in chips was made after workers in Sweden were exposed to an industrial chemical and it turned out that the same traces were also present in people – and their pets. Efforts are being made to remedy the problem, including by cooking at lower temperatures and by genetically engineering an acrylamide-free potato.

It has now been seen that some AGEs can trigger inflammation and that people with diabetes tend to have high counts of them in their blood and bodily systems. While not much is known about specific AGEs, they are not associated with carbohydrates, and diabetics who go on a "low-AGE" diet tend to regain improved insulin sensitivity.

So sugar may be involved in an ultimately deadly mechanism, although it is one driven by cooking and requires a protein to come into existence. Whereas Paleolithic snacks were probably raw foods, the widespread consumption of processed snack foods increases our intake of these glycated products, not least as they continue to form during storage. Scientists have not yet established standards for how to identify, describe, quantify, and test for AGEs, so knowledge is thin. Many big food brands buy in flavoring elements from suppliers in this highly-secretive sector.[16] Different assays have reported quite different results on food mainstays such as cola sodas, olive oil, butter, pasta, and vegetarian dishes.[17]

According to a Danish team that recently conducted a broad review of what is known, AGE formation often relies, alongside the protein's amino acid, on a monosaccharide. But Maillard reactions have been reported even for complex sugars – and in some instances appear to occur spontaneously inside a body that has eaten sugars and fats separately. Different protein sources appear also to have a critical role in the frequency with which AGEs form.[18]

While sugar is needed to galvanize fat to make an AGE, carbohydrates in general are not very involved. That however means that a chunk of the protein we eat is hijacked and if broken down in our lower gut could release products toxic to our organs or deleterious to the epithelial wall separating our gut from our blood supply. In order to understand the mechanics of their effect on human health, what needs to be known is whether these AGEs find a way to crawl into and hijack adipocyte cells and turn abdominal fat into a highly disadvantageous property, as well as what happens to them when they head into the colon and face our microbial warriors there. The question is if and how they are absorbed; it could even be that levels seen in blood plasma are not an ideal indicator if they are hiding out somewhere else rather than being flushed out of our system. The challenge is magnified by their sheer variety.

In the meantime, a team at Mount Sinai Hospital in New York has graciously made an effort to identify where AGEs tend to congregate, using their institution's cafeteria as a base.

In terms of weight, they are very present in meat and salmon when cooked, especially with oil, in fried eggs, French fries, and infant formula. Other curiosities include greater AGE presence in wheat bread than white bread, the sky-high levels reported for olive oil, and that diet colas appears to have quite a lot more than their full-sugar peers. Refined sugar, of course, contains none on its own.[19]

The existence of AGEs links primordial human genius to anxieties about the scale of ultra-processed foods today. Pasta, for example, can be dried at ambient temperature, but that can take up to sixty hours. So today it is usually mixed, kneaded, then extruded and given a short high-temperature drying, which offers major productivity gains – plus more than 300 shapes – and several desirable shelf-life traits. At the same time, it opens the door, however modestly, for AGEs.

The same is the case for *torrefacto* coffee, popular in Spain and Argentina, which involves tossing some sugar on coffee beans in the roasting process. That protects the beans from oxidation, although some suspect it began as a way to hide poor-quality beans. The pretzel is another love-child of the process, as it came about when a Bavarian baker accidentally used caustic soda instead of sugar water as a glaze, and customers liked it.

To be sure, the Maillard reaction has offered abundant pleasure over time – and it is common for dinner guests to applaud their host's ability to produce it. "It should be called the flavor reaction," says Nathan Myrhvold, founder of Seattle-based Modernist Cuisine, a group that has "R&D chefs" and the kind of high-tech kitchen laboratory you'd expect from Microsoft's former chief technology officer. He doesn't sound worried. But more research will have to be done, especially after an important recent experiment found that wild-type mice given high-AGE diets – "thermally processed nutrients" – not only developed insulin resistance but that their progeny eventually developed it shortly after birth as the result of precociously eroded defense mechanisms.

It took only three generations for what Weijing Cai, the lead scientist and based at Mount Sinai School of Medicine, called a "phenotypic shift" towards obesity, adiposity, and insulin resistance to occur. "These changes replicate the metabolic syndrome phenotype that is becoming increasingly common in adult humans," and only sustained restriction of the oxidant food supply of our industrial society can allow for the restoration of lost gene function and "restore native resistance" to diabetes and other chronic diseases including Alzheimer's disease, Cai said.[20]

A recent study supports that view, as overweight Danish women put on a low-AGE diet had better insulin sensitivity within a month. That said, while the pace and determinants of AGEs accumulation in the body are largely unknown, there is strong evidence that they form faster in situations of oxidative stress or persistent hyperglycemia.[21]

Cai's third-generation observation is a concern given the increase in pediatric obesity, for today's kids are the grandkids of people who grew up at time when major food-processing techniques, some developed during the war effort, were rolled out. The prospect that our demise is due to the hyperindustrialization of cooking, which made our species what it is, may prove scarier than any epidemic.

Gut Reaction

5

By digestibility of food several things are, or may be, meant.

Wilbur Olin Atwater[1]

It turns out that the catchall phrase "you are what you eat" is not entirely true. For decades, nutritional scientists have operated with an in-out model, weighing and measuring what people eat and then weighing and measuring – for trace calories and details about them – what we excrete. The difference was our energy intake, which we either used or turned into fat.

One of the exciting scientific fields today suggests that in fact we always have company for dinner, even when we snack at our desks. They are the rowdy inhabitants of our gut, our microbiome.

"We really need to think of ourselves as a superorganism," says Liping Zhao, professor of microbiology at Shanghai Jiao Tong University and one of the world leaders in the study of the ancient beings we host in an outsourcing deal struck long ago that allows us to focus on thinking while handing over the keys to our large intestine.

Scientists had for some time suspected that gut bacteria were busy, and more than a century ago a biologist first remarked on how one particular strain was prevalent in infants, but the advent of high throughput sequencing, used to map the human genome and allowing the relatively rapid genetic identification of large numbers of microorganisms, has revolutionized understanding in recent years and pointed to dramatically different causal mechanisms between what we eat and our health.

The human microbiome resides mostly in the lower intestine – remember, ours are shorter than those of our primate cousins – and specifically near and on our mucosal tissues. Between us and them is a slim single layer of epithelium, the 400-square-meter gut wall that is quite literally our last line of defense as what passes through enters our bloodstream. Just how many critters live down there remains unknown, but it's pretty certain that they vastly outnumber us. The canonical comparison, cited in countless research papers, has been that our bodies have 10 trillion cells and provide refuge to ten times as many microbes, but the source of that number was recently tracked down to the examination in 1972 of a single gram of human fecal matter.[2]

Bacteria, viruses, fungi, and other microorganisms have long been seen as unwelcome vectors of plague, typhoid and other germ-based diseases, and so the only good bug was a dead one, and the pharmaceutical industry has prospered making agents to kill the evil pathogens. It would be foolish to rain on the parade of antibiotics as perhaps the greatest triumph of the human sciences.

Now, however, we're learning that the denizens of our murky gut biota do us a number of favors in their dark and airless space, such as help send signals to our brains that affect and perhaps dictate everything from our mood and intelligence to our susceptibility to disease. Some of them even pay rent by acting as soldiers against invading pathogens we mistakenly ingest, which means they are armed.

We are essentially germ-free until birth, when we inhale microbes as we traverse through the vaginal passage, thereby receiving as an endowment our mother's microbiome regime in one giant big bang. Some more come upon breastfeeding, including precious *Bifidobacteria* transmitted from complex sugars in maternal milk. While there is much to know, this original endowment acts as a personal trainer for our immune system from the get go. It is specially designed in anticipation of our likely nutritional environment and promulgates a first division between dietary friends and foes.

While we come into contact with microbes all the time, even by using cutlery and furniture and breathing, the gut biota tends to be remarkably conservative. Indeed, a new study has found 80 percent of our other selves can be uniquely identified as ours a year after we leave them somewhere as microbial "fingerprints."[3]

While extremely resilient, microbiomes can change. Antibiotics, for example, can create regime shifts, pummeling one species and so indirectly favoring another. That is one reason why severe diarrhea-causing and dehydrating infections by *Clostridium difficile* bacteria so often occur in hospitals, as they claw their way into an undefended space. Another way to change the gut biota is via fecal transplant, a stool transfer meant to tweak and bolster diversity. So far, these are often done between family members, so continuity remains substantial and the transplant aims merely at reversing a recent imbalance between bacterial species.[4] The US FDA claims regulatory purview over this novel "drug" while it reviews the procedure's growing clinical use.

After the maternal endowment, diet is the predominant pathway for microbiota to develop. This is not so much because new bacteria hitchhike in on the food we eat as because what we consume offers differing stimuli to who we already have as guests, stoking exuberant growth of one or another species – which tend to hang out in different niches along our digestive tract.

The reason we are talking about this in a book about sugar is because "sweetness and light" was meant to mean bringing the best of human knowledge to bear on any subject. In this case, the burgeoning scientific field has quickly identified that the microbiome can be upset, giving rise to what is formally known as "dysbiosis" and often takes the specific outward forms of obesity and Type 2 diabetes.

In short, the heavyweight problem once blamed on animal fats and now so often blamed on excess added sugar may not stem from what we eat, but on whether our commensal friends are thriving or starving.

As there are so many microbes to identify – and they are usually hard to culture separately as their trademark feature is to live in environments without oxygen – there is much scientists do not know. On the other hand, as Zhao, who is also director of two Shanghai laboratories specializing in ecogenomics and nutrition, says, progress in teasing out the real nature of these critters is moving very fast.

Obesity, it turns out, is a big reason for that. Time and time again researchers have found that a fecal transplant from a lean donor has a dramatic effect on an obese one. That can backfire. In early 2015, doctors in Rhode Island reported on a 32-year-old woman patient who had been having chronic abdominal pain that serial antibiotic treatments did not alleviate. The woman, who was healthy, had a BMI of 26, and weighed 136 pounds, opted to receive a fecal transplant from her teenage daughter, who had a BMI of 26.4 that turned out to be rising. That did the trick for her pain, but sixteen months later she had put on 34 pounds and had a BMI of 34.5 – despite exercising, forswearing sugary drinks and even trying a liquid protein diet monitored by specialists.[5]

What happened in that case has been documented systematically in laboratory rats. The breakthrough paper on the subject – which helped catalyze the deluge of ongoing microbiota research – was published in 2005, when Ruth Ley and her colleagues raised sets of mice born from parents genetically programmed to be obese alongside another set of wild-type rodents and a third hybrid set. The former proved true to form and grew fat. Upon dissection, they revealed guts with only half as many as the wild-type mouselets, and a mirror increase in *Firmicutes*.[6] These are the two largest groups of bacteria in the gut, and scientists were initially excited about a possible B:F ratio predicting an overweight-prone gut typology. A 20 percent shift from one to the other – which is easily plausible to judge by genome sequences reported so far – may represent an unwitting capacity to harvest an extra 150 calories from our daily diet, equal to that can of Coca-Cola in New York's anti-soda campaign, according to one recent study.[7]

Another early landmark *Bacteroidetes* breakthrough found that germ-free mice fed an ad libitum high-sugar, high-fat diet did not put on any extra weight at all, although they did after being "conventionalized" with the transplanted gut biota of an obese mouse. That further indicated the potentially vast alchemy of the intestinal underworld, showing it went beyond energy harvesting and has a signaling role in our neuro-immunological circuits.[8]

"Our intestinal microbiota is an integral part of ourselves and cross-talk between the intestinal microbiota and host leads to life-long epigenetic programming," which is an all-new approach to "so-called 'lifestyle' diseases," says Karen Scott, a scientist at the Rowett Institute of Nutrition and Health in Aberdeen, Scotland.[9] The new insights cast fresh light on an observation made in an earlier obesity outbreak in the nineteenth century by Charles Bouchard, a French doctor who observed that less than half of his obese patients actually ate too much, and some of them grew overweight even though they didn't eat enough.[10]

The enthusiasm is palpable, and one experiment has now been successfully done in which ordinary laboratory mice were treated with antibiotics to turn their colon into a blank slate and then given a new microbiome, which successfully set up shop. While there is much to learn about the ideal timing of such a maneuver, its potential application to create a standard for humans is self-evident and the authors explicitly note that the idea of their method is to "humanize" the gut of animal models.[11]

Justin Sonnenberg, another star in this field from Stanford University, thinks the microbiome should be seen as a technology platform for human health and many suspect the services it is already offering influence an array of diseases known as or related to metabolic syndrome.

In this case, the mice carrying the obese human microbiome ended up housing more of the microbial genes involved in stress responses and detoxification, and promptly showed symptoms typical of an obese, insulin-sensitive human. Recipients of the lean endowment, by contrast, had higher expression of microbial genes involved in the digestion of plant-derived polysaccharides – complex fibers – and other processes associated with happy metabolism.[12] Then, in what could be seen as a sociological survey, they let all the animals cohabit to see if microbes might hop from one body to another. Mice are coprophagic, meaning they eat excrement, and so, it turned out that the fat mouselets that hung out with the lean ones put on less weight – and gained immigrant *Bacteroidetes* – than the obese ones which kept to themselves. To round off the exercise, they found that when they were given a menu full of fruit and vegetables with less fat, the obese mice still gained more weight than the lean ones.

One has an almost foreboding sense that causality, that elusive holy grail for the reams of correlation-based observational hypotheses rolled out by those seeking to indict sugar, is finally at hand – and that looking for culpable foods has been barking up the wrong tree.

So what about mice and men?

It's not going to be easy. While reports that mice carrying human microbes and switched to a high-fat, high-sugar diet can undergo microbiota regime changes in a single day, making the trick work the other way appears more difficult, and even more so in humans who are more diverse than off-the-rack germ-free mice. A survey of 154 humans, mostly twins and their mothers, did not produce a single bacterial species in common that was meaningfully present.

All that points to environmental conditions playing a substantial role, or as researchers put it, "the phylogenetic tree of bacterial life in the gut consists primarily of shallow twigs" and that, rather than setting down strong root systems like a tree does in soil, "the gut selects for diversification in the few deep evolutionary lineages that flourish there."[13]

Still, it turns out that men with metabolic syndrome given smidgens of microbiomial mass from lean donors saw their peripheral insulin sensitivity improved within six weeks. Dutch researchers have reported that the median rate of glucose disappearance, a proxy for how our bodies handle insulin, rose by more than 60 percent on average after the infusion.[14]

Scientists, often working in large international teams to carry out the genomic computations, have since compared the intestinal populations of rural Africans and urban Finns, fat and thin people from the same city, and a host of other provocative comparisons. Two bacterial types have been identified as prospective anti-obesity warriors, but it's not yet clear what makes things tick. It is more likely that diversity itself constitutes metabolic magic, and for the record Americans host the fewest microbial species.

The foregoing examples suggest that it may one day be possible to dismantle metabolic syndrome, not through dietary and behavioral regulations but through the strategic deployment rather than the elimination of germs.[15] The obesity epidemic may in fact not be about excess but absence. Apologies will be due!

Look at it another way

Would policy support for state intervention through dietary rules such as mandatory sugar reduction change if the cause of the problem, identified as the risk of obesity and non-communicative diseases that often accompany it, were understood to be linked to the microbiome instead of parts of the food system?

It may be. Let's look at the question in an awkwardly personal way.

It turns out that mice born naturally have a more robust set of intestinal bacteria, and a better immune system, than those born by C-section. Danish biologists tracked mice of each kind from birth, noticing they each had different gut flora at the beginning of their lives but converged over the longer term. The poorer immune system of the latter mice persisted, however, as if it had been installed as an operating system. The naturally born mice had more regulatory T-cells, dubbed "tregs", which militate against the risk that a body attacks part of itself or something it needs, such as insulin, which normally serves as a signaling device to the brain about energy allocation and consequent food intake.[16]

In this case, we too are a bit mousy. Dozens of recent studies have found that children born via C-section are very significantly more likely to have trouble with overweight, asthma, and diabetes later. Delivery by C-section was associated with a 46 percent higher risk of obesity already during childhood according to a recent study of 436 mothers in New York form 1998 through 2006.[17]

Children exposed to antibiotics during the second or third trimester of their pregnancy had an 84 percent higher risk of obesity compared to those not so exposed, according to the same study. That would be tantamount to truckloads of extra sugar.

In Canada, a study found that babies born via C-section and thus skipping the traditional endowment of their mother's microbiome, often ended up short of *Bacteroidetes* and other bacteria that help set up house and serve as a welcoming committee – or guard dog – for future arrivals. And that is happening around the world. When such infrastructure is underdeveloped, the immune system's policing instinct often overreacts, triggering inflammation responses even for trivial reasons.

Asthma is more likely. So is obesity. And so, apparently, is the sensitivity to gluten that has spurred a large market in alternative grain-based foods in the past decade. Childhood-onset diabetes, known as Type 1, is 20 percent more likely, according to a set of international studies.[18]

The huge increase in C-sections around the world is thus cause for some concern. While the microbiome has not been completely mapped or understood, medical professionals are convinced the lack of a big-gulp natural birth passage is a critical missing link. After all, the epithelial wall is the largest surface area of the human body exposed to the environment.

Because C-sections are common and often a matter of choice rather than need, public health officials hasten to say there may be other reasons, including latent genetic factors, and that the cause of these correlations is yet unknown. Moreover, C-sections are often required because mothers are obese, raising the specter of a doomsday loop.

It is widely known that new mothers often report difficulty breastfeeding after a C-section and turn to formula, the quintessence of refined carbohydrates. That means missing a phase where the nearly magical sugars of a mother's milk further fortifiy their infant's intestinal friends by fostering *Bifidobacteria*, a species that appears beneficial and may help coach the immune system in its early days. While our microbiome is largely set up over the first three years of life, the evidence points to the importance of a sequence, starting with ample *Bifidobacteria* and introducing fibers for *Bacteroidetes* and the other bacterial types later. "Basic laboratory based research is supplementing the epidemiologic studies," says Joseph Neu, a professor of pediatrics at the University of Florida.[19] That's a sober methodological observation.

Martin Blaser, director of the Human Biome Institute at New York University, proffers a more urgent, nearly moral tone. "The aggregate of modern assaults on the early life microbiome suggests that our progeny may not be inheriting their fair share," he writes.[20]

So is the C-section baby a modern-day version of the infant falling into London's River Thames in the Hogarth print discussed earlier? That child was quite likely that of an affluent socialite who had hired the drunken woman as a wet nurse.

There is no doubt that the number of C-section births has skyrocketed; it has risen from 4.5 percent in the USA in 1965 to 32.7 percent today, risen fourfold since the 1970s in enlightened Norway, is now close to half in China – even in the countryside – and a hefty 80 percent in some private clinics in Brazil, where one major hospital recently set up strict daytime hours for childbirth. In Europe, there's a sharp regional divide, with single-digit rates in Nordic countries and higher rates in the south, peaking at 52 percent for Cyprus.

The WHO has repeatedly suggested it be kept below 15 percent, saying there is no evidence that mortality rates rise when a national C-section goes above 10 percent. Its white papers on the subject focus primarily not on health but on the correlation between rising incomes and more frequent C-sections, warning that the procedure weighs too heavily on health care budgets.[21]

It is of course a woman's choice, but it may also be part of the obesity epidemic.[22]

Given the draconian health risks[23] it poses for the newborn, and its highly-corroborated association with obesity via the microbiome, it is striking that the nutritional police are not on the warpath. One wonders whether that may in any way reflect the political style preferred by many of the people who engage in policy reform activism. Cultural factors, many reflecting discretionary incentives, appear to be a major driving force – quite possibly larger than any other – in the increase of C-sections.

Whereas poor dietary choices are often associated with the poor, the C-section has more of an elite feel. It's a delicate matter. Some reports say voluntary C-sections comprise less than 3 percent of US births. Given that 80 percent of C-sections in that country are considered low risk, this would imply that almost all of the others represent hospital insistence, be it to rationalize work schedules, take in higher fees, or ward off potential litigation. Many people today may not even know whether they were born by C-section and would certainly be shocked to be told that, with their compromised microbiome, they are at higher risk of obesity or diabetes. Many might also object to the idea that, just as obese people have been criticized for undisciplined gluttony and flawed lifestyles, they are now responsible for putting their own children on a trajectory with an unhappy destiny. Maybe a judge will one day have to decide.

The science now collides with a well-entrenched view that the whole matter cannot even be allowed as a subject for public health and policy concern. In Connecticut, affluent parents were appalled when a local kindergarten required parents of prospective students to indicate how their child was born, claiming that was an invasion of privacy over what should be the jurisdiction of the individual. Milan daily *Corriere della Sera* expressed bemused horror at America's rigid ways, omitting to mention that at 38 percent, Italy's C-section rate is the second-highest in Europe.

Privacy concerns are always commendable. But do they hold up in a real epidemic?

Elite social concerns may be put to the test on this point. The voluntary rate for C-sections is almost certainly far higher than the oft-repeated figure noted earlier, reflecting the simple fact that such data is not formally collected. A review of highly-detailed actual patient data at Yale University's hospital found that maternal-request C-sections were three times higher than the canonically quoted figure and rising at a 27 percent annual rate, faster than any other kind.[24]

The same is evidently the case in Europe, as indicated by the huge variation in obstetricians' self-reported willingness to offer a surgical delivery upon request in an uncomplicated pregnancy. That ranges from nearly 80 percent in the UK and Germany, down to only 15 percent in Spain, in theory showing a strong role for national cultural and religious traits and perhaps legal liability regimes. Gender and age of medical staff may also matter – for example, Italian obstetricians were far more likely to be male than British ones, and they were six times more likely to be over the age of 50.[25]

But what people say often amounts to empty calories. Spanish doctors, for example, claim to be the least likely to accept a maternal request, but somewhere along the line they apparently relent as the country has one of Europe's highest C-section rates. It's hard to imagine what a policy debate would mean without recognizing what's happening in the world of practice.

While developing countries face much higher maternal mortality rates and many births occur at home, the clinical situation in their formal sectors appears to be driven by similar trends. A thumping 49 percent of births at the Muhimbili National Hospital in Tanzania's capital city are by C-section today. Most of the mothers who go there do so of their own volition, and many have private health insurance, indicating fairly affluent social backgrounds.[26]

Evidence that C-sections are culturally perceived as "more elegant and modern" abounds in many fast-growing economies such as China – where the military now worries its recruits are too pudgy to fit into army tanks – and Brazil, where thousands of extra-wide seats had to be added to World Cup stadiums in line with national laws that infrastructure cater to the special needs of the disabled, including the one in six adults in the country now classified as obese.

The people of Brazil, a country of 200 million that has eradicated hunger and joined the ranks of middle-income nations in the past generation, offer a special example of the role of culture in global trends. Brazilian immigrants to Portugal are 50 percent more likely than any other group in the country – including immigrants from Angola, another former colony – to undergo C-sections, even after adjusting for a slew of factors such as age and income. Brazilian immigrants in Norway and Finland also opt for C-sections at more than twice the rate of local women.

Investigating that perplexity, Christina Texeira, an epidemiologist at the University of Porto, found no other reason than culture – namely that a C-section was a symbol of high status. As the free national health service does not formally recognize maternal requests for C-sections, Brazilians in Portugal must have used forceful social signaling methods to obtain such a high rate, she adds.[27]

Beauty is evidently a subject of some pressure in Brazil, where women are three times more likely to describe themselves as beautiful than their Portuguese peers – and are also four times more likely to have considered cosmetic surgery! – according to a survey commissioned by Dove, a beauty products company. They were also far more likely to consider body weight, hair style, youthfulness, sexiness, and financial success – all factors that may have had a lesser role in indigenous communities – as critical factors in being beautiful.[28]

Interestingly, Mexican immigrants in the USA – who are more likely to come from an indigenous background than Brazilians – behave in the opposite way, notably compared to Latino people who emigrated long before, also suggesting a strong attachment to their culture of origin.[29] Meanwhile, a graphic mapping of obesity rates over time shows a striking correlation with the rise of the C-section, far sharper than that of the sugar supply, and science has now grasped the plausible causal link.

In landmark research published in the prestigious British medical journal *The Lancet* in 2014, no fewer than 141 authors collaborated to find that the worldwide prevalence of overweight and obesity rose by half to 41.7 percent from 1980 and 2013, which when factoring in population growth meant a near tripling of individuals to 2.1 billion. Citing changes in the gut microbiome as a potential factor, they noted that the most rapid growth was in people aged 20 to 40 in developing countries while also emphasizing a striking increase among young people in developed countries.[30]

Adding a lag time of twenty years to let newborns mature, it would appear the above trend fits nicely with the expanded use of C-sections, which began in earnest after the 1960s with the development of anesthesias. Ironically, the surgical techniques had been mostly perfected in the late 1800s to cope with an epidemic surge in rickets – a vitamin deficiency once attributed to diet but later understood to be caused by lack of sunlight as rapidly industrializing Europe drew droves of people into urban slums. One of the key functions we've outsourced to our microbiome is the handling of vitamin D.

The point of this interlude is to ask why the anti-obesity crusaders urging policy-makers to take regulatory action against a specific food –

demon sugar, in this case, but it has been fat and on current form could one day be corn or wheat or tomatoes – are not so vocal on this.

The reasons seem eminently social and cultural. So does much of what drives the campaign to insist a common food causes disease.

A flashlight in the *selva oscura*

"The human microbiome works like a rain forest," Zhao says. "Its foundation species are like the trees that form a canopy which, once the forest is complete, cover and encompass a very unique environment." He adds: "If you remove a keystone species, it all collapses."

So, sorry to say, there is no ideal microbiome. After all, people have different cultures and have lived in extremely different alimentary environments, ranging from Inuit communities living mostly on animal fat to Pacific islanders running up massive cholesterol levels thanks to heavy reliance on coconuts, and neither suffering particularly adverse health consequences.

That does not mean, however, that there won't be major therapeutic breakthroughs. In fact, Zhao is currently engaged in an ongoing practical experiment with 21 Chinese kids born with Prader-Willi syndrome (PBS), an obesity-inducing genetic condition affecting around one in 15,000 people. The syndrome causes a host of problems including extremely weak muscle tone and hyperphagia, or severe overeating due to an uncontrollable feeling of hunger. It typically leads to restricted cognitive skills and compulsive behavior such as lying, stealing, scavenging, and eating even frozen foods. People with PBS do not go through puberty, pharmaceutical potions have been tried in vain, and many end up relying on growth hormones to boost stature while taking behavior-controlling drugs.

The research team did an analysis of their gut biota and found they were broadly similar to ordinary obese peers. So they subjected the kids, some of them weighing 60 kilograms or 130 pounds at the age of five, along with 21 obese children without the faulty gene, to three months of a balanced diet with ample helpings of traditional Chinese medicinal foods and prebiotics as well as non-digestible but fermentable carbohydrates and phytochemicals designed to shake things up in the intestine. All responded with notable weight loss, improved metabolic signals, less inflammation – the trigger for most disorders – and increased counts of *Bifidobacteria*.

One of the volunteers shed 58 kilograms in nine months and went on of his own accord to halve his weight to 73 kilograms, after eighteen months of this diet, without any particular exercise regime at all, while the others lost on average 19 percent of their weight in three months.

For an empirical check, Zhao then infused their original microbiomes into germ-free mice, who bloated up, and then took the later microbiome from the same individual, whereupon the mice did not become fat. "Something must have happened," Zhao laconically observed.

Because his team was interested in precisely what that was. In line with his emphasis on the rain forest canopy, Zhao insisted on analyzing bacterial genomics at the level of the strain rather than the genus or even higher taxonomic rank. He thinks the idea of a B:F master ratio is primitive, and it is bacterial functions rather than their genetic class that makes the microbiome tick. The microbiome is a whole, and can be pathogenic or not. When he looked closer, what he found violates much of what modern nutritional thought is based on. Gut bacteria typically take undigested food, extract protein and energy for themselves, and send the rest on to the liver, which prepares it for excretion. That much is broadly known. But by searching more than 2 million gut genes and comparing them to both urinary metabolites and the genes in the original food sources to identify specific enzymes engaged in activities that might have led to the changed microbiome regime, the Shanghai team located bacterial entities that, instead of gorging on carbohydrates for energy, began gobbling up proteins – and sending elements to the liver that processed it and emitted agents known to spur increased adiposity.[31]

"Why were they doing that?" Zhao wondered, noting that organisms are supposed to use carbohydrates for energy and use protein to grow. The answer, he concluded, is that the bacteria were basically starving. "They didn't have enough carbohydrates, and their only available nutrient was protein, so they tried to use that for energy," he said.

There's a reason athletes chow down on pasta or high-carbohydrate meals before their performance, and save the prime rib for later. It lets them maximize, in time for the game, the energy their body takes in. Eating a steak before the game would make one a bit groggy on the pitch. The bacteria Zhao was watching faced a similar predicament, and their life was at stake. Only some species are likely to manage the trick. The ones that do will thrive and send on the unoxidized part of their energy source to the liver, one of whose tasks is to metabolize nitrogen and convert it into glucose to be released into the blood. Excessive amounts of this leads to high blood glucose, the diabetic signature trait.

So if the bad-guy bacteria are living off protein, should we cut back on meat and legumes? Should we further ramp up our carbohydrate consumption to encourage the critters to behave better? The lesson of the microbiome is: no, and sort of.

"Gut bacteria need not be beneficial, they just need to eat," Zhao said. The real issue is that the denizens of the lower intestine were not being fed, and those that learned how to make shift anyway had adverse effects on their human hosts' regulatory systems. In short, if they start cannibalizing protein for energy, it's not because there is too much protein, but rather not enough of the kind of carbohydrates they like – the fibrous ones we can't digest.

Mutualistic relationships require complementarity, so when parties start acting similarly, elaborate structures of reciprocity break down and are replaced by cut-throat competition. That sounds like a dystopian description of what happens when societies move from close-knit, face-to-face village communities to the big anonymous capitalist city, but we're still talking about how we eat here.

People need energy, and there are more of us today, so we have become increasingly efficient at reaping it where we can. Highly-processed carbohydrate foods – and yes, refined sugar is included in this large supermarket category – allow humans to obtain ample energy without leaving leftovers, triggering downstream starvation. It's not about skipping dessert but about not skipping salad.

Perhaps our modern food system is making us act like the C4 plants. A fire burns down a forest, grasses take over, and, well, we graze. By adapting, we ward off our own extinction. Gut bacteria are no different. Altered microbiomes don't want to go back to the old ways, so when individuals have metabolic problems, they are hard to fix, according to Zhao. The newly populous gut bacteria with a taste for protein as an energy source they use somewhat wastefully protest when their lifestyle is put at risk. They need to be countered by fostering beneficial bacterial populations, and feeding them appropriately.

To be drastic, one could compare them to shadow bankers using short-term value-at-risk models for mortgage bonds that keep validating themselves so long as house prices rise. It works until it doesn't. Then a big systemic bailout is needed and authorities huddle to find a way to regulate a sector that is broken. Such things can happen.

But it would be wrong to lump bankers all together. By boring below the level of bacterial species to focus on specific strains, Zhao found a world that gave rise to his metaphor of the rain forest. It turns out that species can form ad hoc alliances with others to produce roving bands – he calls them "guilds" – to adapt to environmental changes. A bacterial type does not have a single assigned function. They aren't nationalist, as it were.

That flexibility also means that the way bacterial cohorts interact can change dramatically, leading at times to paradoxical situations similar to how, when a grazing animal is eliminated from an ecosystem, the grass does not prosper but fire and desertification ensues.

In their experiment, which identified 18 such guilds in each person's gut, a genome interaction group containing Bifidobacterium species rose to predominance, muscling out the guild that had previously housed the toxin-producing bugs.

Zhao thinks the good guild identified above may point the way to the existence of a foundation species in the human microbiome, the tree supporting the rain forest canopy as it were, and as such a primary target for supportive interventions from outside. Even if so, effective treatments for obesity, be they pharmaceutical drugs or nutritional prebiotics, will require identifying both the unwanted species and then locating – as a target – the functional guild to which it belongs.

To put it in popular foodie terms, it is akin to realizing that olive oil is not the secret sauce of the Mediterranean diet but rather the proxy for the inclusion of a lot of raw plants and fibers.

In a broad sense, Zhao says his research shows that the problem of obesity is not what we eat, but what we do *not* eat: non-digestible carbohydrates that can be fermented by the gut bacteria, with a splash of phytochemicals. These were increased eightfold, to 49 grams a day, for the kids in the Shanghai experiment. That's equal to 14 cups of raw spinach, or 25 bowls of Wheaties cereal!

Scientific innovation based on millions of genetic computations, then, brings us back to the usual prescription: eat more dietary fiber, more fruits and vegetables. Whole grains are okay, and ketchup is better than mayonnaise on your burger, red wine is recommended, but bigger bonuses can be reaped from foods such as onions, broccoli, berries, and especially herbs like mint – and it's often the chemicals they carry within them that are the key element.[32] These are the fibers that we personally don't seem to need, but are bribes to convince germs to do things we want.

In a world of nutritional spin, it is sensible to be clear about what we mean by fiber, a word that is casually tossed around on food blogs and in ordinary conversation. The strict view is that the word should refer to non-starch intrinsic plant cell-wall polysaccharides. That is, parts of actual plants. The broad and more functionalist view is that fiber means anything that passes through the small intestine unscathed. The difference is substantial and explains the controversy over whether sugars naturally occurring in fruit should be deemed to be different from refined sugar, which is a proverbially huge sticking point in discussions about recommended sugar levels, as nobody wants to criticize fresh fruit.

The stricter definition, endorsed by and wonderfully explained by Klaus Englyst, refers to chemical elements, polysaccharides such as inulin, that have a structural function in the integrity of the cells and tissues of a living organism, in particular giving fruit and vegetables their ability to hold high amounts of water, which is the main reason they are calorie-light when measured in bulk. Other nutrition-salient elements can be synthesized to be indigestible, but they don't have that legacy, which means they also don't have the natural trace elements – phytochemicals and micronutrients – that the former likely acquired. Call it *terroir*, to use a wine-lover's term.

Englyst notes that the dietary benefits of fiber may not be so much their texture and slow-release of energy as the small amounts of precious elements they carry with them.[33] Hence whole grains are superior in health terms not only because they retain the germ and bran fractions removed in the refining process, but also because they contain phytochemical traces. The virtues of fiber may actually lie in the company it keeps.

This explains why honey, which is around 90 percent sucrose, is often hailed as a health food even by those who scoff at sugar. Honey contains many different types of polysaccharides that – we now can grasp – are highly appreciated in our lower intestine and stoke species richness.[34]

Meanwhile, Cargill, the agrochemical giant, has invented Oliggo-Fiber inulin, a soluble fiber derived from the chicory root for food processors to incorporate into their products. It's a powder hailed for having little taste that can invisibly add in nutrition. It is even available in liquid form, so there is now such a thing in our food system as a "fiber syrup."

Here's the thing: all that is good, in that it adds inulin, a known beneficial substance, and helps cover our fiber deficit. Still, it is highly unlikely that Cargill's engineers can match the enigmatic way bees acquire ecological exposure and add it to their honey, nor for that matter the similar skills of traditional medicinal plants identified by human cultures over many generations.

Microbiome science will likely now be able to discover which synthetic products work. Consider Olestra, designed to be a calorie-free fat and pave the way to guilt-free Pringles with no impact on one's girth. It is an engineered product with a sucrose core caged in by edible oils that was actually discovered during a search for a way to help fatten up premature babies. It's essentially a plastic, and shoots through the small intestine to the large one. It thus counts as a dietary fiber – and is classified as one by the FDA.

On the other hand, Olestra suffered a publicity problem linked to alleged flatulence – not the first fiber to be so accused – and while it does what it says on the package, it also has a tendency to absorb vitamins on its way through the gut, making it a bit of a mechanical pathogen. People who eat a lot of Pringles may also have a lot of apparent fat in their feces – out of the body, as was the point – a common symptom of pancreatic dysfunction, but that's a problem regarding diagnosis rather than food.

Is it a food? Some decry Olestra as a symbol of reductionist nutritionism. Still, the opportunities are there. Other projects, such as the EU's "Nutra-Snacks" initiative, aim to find a more organic product. The challenge there is that it's still hard to know which phytochemicals one wants in it, and achieving production scale is elusive.

It's complex. But two things are clear. First, nutritional knowledge is itself a kind of fiber and will both influence and be reworked by the microbiome. And second, the missing part of the western obesogenic diet is not huge; a shift of 3 or 4 percent of our daily intake may restore the metabolic rift.

So you can chow down, probably even ad libitum, so long as you set up a foraging mechanism to bring you phytochemicals and other tasteless wonders. "You can eat as much sugar as you want, or drink as many sodas, as long as you take in enough of the nondigestible carbs," says Zhao. Sugar is just calories, which we need. The problem of the modern diet that has triggered the metabolic alarms, he says, is not any single food, but forgetting to eat the stuff we can't digest. Highly-processed foods are a concern because we keep all their energy benefit to ourselves, which is rude.

Ordinary sugar has not turned up as a problem food in the gut research so far, probably because it is digested before making it to the lower intestine. But non-caloric artificial sweeteners, saccharin, and sucralose – all of which naturally are not digested and so travel to the lower intestine – were shown to induce alterations to the microbiome that lead to glucose intolerance when consumed in large doses by mice and humans.[35]

Two commonly used emulsifiers, carboxymethyl cellulose, often labeled E-466 and found in candy and cottage cheese as well as toothpaste, and polysorbate-80, often found in cosmetics, vitamins, and pharmaceutical products, also appeared to trigger bacterial perturbations leading to higher bile acid levels that reduce the thickness of the epithelial wall when given in fairly low doses to mice. More tests will have to be done, on these and other food additives, many of which have never been investigated in terms of their impact on intestinal bacteria.[36]

To each their own

While on the cusp of major breakthroughs in our understanding of our world, microbiome research represents an important paradigm shift of the kind that often emerges when problems are analyzed dynamically as ecosystems instead of approached in the hope of finding a reductionist and universal rule. We are all, after all, guild members.

Excitement over potential therapeutic discoveries linked to the microbiome is strong and research is expanding across the board. We now know how piglet guts change if they forage on chicory, a great source of inulin, the kind of prebiotic that *Bifidobacteria* love and which has fallen out of the modern food system. And we even know that 26 percent of the bacterial species in US municipal sewage systems come from humans, which may one day give health officials advance warning of where metabolic troubles are brewing.

More troublingly, we also know that iron-fortified maize porridge for Kenyan infants, recommended to combat anemia, significantly raised the number of pathogenic bacteria in their guts, triggering severe diarrhea, the world's second leading cause of death for children under the age of five.[37]

As Zhao's notion of roving bands highlights, the microbiome isn't a ticket to utopia and there is no right formula. But when our gut bacteria revolt and punch holes in our epithelial wall, we know that's a bad one.

With so many diseases of affluence in modern societies, there has also been particular interest in the possible virtues to be found in the microbiomes of people living in less developed countries. Italian researchers, led by Carlotta De Filippo of the University of Florence, led a project to compare the microbiota of European children and their peers in rural Burkina Faso, presumed to have a high-fiber diet similar to that of "early human settlements at the time of the birth of agriculture."

After DNA sequencing and biochemical analyses on the scat they collected, they found a low B:F ratio prevailed in Africa – which readers by now might have expected – but also an abundance of bacteria from the genuses *Prevotella* and *Xylanibacter.* These organisms specialize in chomping down stuff like plant cellulose, pointing to a likely co-evolution with their hosts, who were thereby able to maximize energy intake from fibers and elude inflammation and other colonic diseases. Both were completely lacking in the kids from Florence, who predictably had high B:F ratios, reflecting consumption of animal fats.

Briefly, the children in Burkina Faso, who were breastfed to the age of 2, mostly ate homegrown millet and sorghum with legumes, often ground and cooked into a thick porridge, along with vegetables and legumes and a slight amount of animal protein in the form of chicken or termites. Their peers in Florence ate more meat, sugar, and fat and their caloric intake was about 50 percent higher at every stage from age 1 to 6, while their fiber intake was roughly half.[38]

The respective B:F ratios reflected "profound differences between the two groups," with 58 percent of the Burkina Faso gut bacteria flying the *Bacteroidetes* flag compared to only 22 percent in Florence and a similar asymmetry in the other direction for *Firmicutes.* General biodiversity was much higher in Africa, which the authors attribute partly to the European consumption of sugar.

The researchers also noted far higher levels of short-chain fatty acids in the Burkina Faso samples, and they surmise that a diet low in sugar and fat would select for bacteria that produce these. They protect against inflammation, which is how adiposity and metabolic ailments get started. On the other hand, they also found that many of these short-chain fatty acids were excreted.

So, while the Burkina Faso kids share generously with their gut, their efficiency in converting food into human energy is lower than the Europeans. Precisely this has long appeared to be one of the major tradeoffs built into the battle for nutritional health. On the one hand, biodiversity increasingly appears to be a practically infinitely good thing, and that's also true for the gut. Indeed, important studies in France and Denmark found that the microbiome gene count was 40 percent smaller in obese people than healthy ones in the same city. As certain bacterial strains appear to be signals of ultimate gut complexity, testing for them could become a useful predictive tool for doctors. Greater gene variety was linked with less body fat, cholesterol, and highly sensitive C-reactive protein, which is commonly sought in blood tests and linked to inflammation.[39]

On the other hand, while global obesity is rising, even in Africa, the continent has an ongoing struggle with undernutrition and the number of hungry people continues to grow.[40] The Burkina Faso diet is healthy, as it were, but woefully low in calories. Indeed, the intake reported for the children is not far above the basal metabolic rate required to keep bodily organs functioning.[41]

Yet the Burkina Faso microbiome militates against adequate energy intake, and while its people are safeguarded from chronic diseases, weak economic output means they are vulnerable to more immediate ones. Subsistence farming may itself be a metabolic regime, in which people can't grow more food because they don't have enough energy due to the low levels of calories they are eating. This is exactly the bind that Europe escaped, starting with an agricultural productivity revolution in England that eventually led to colonial trade and ever-increasing imports of dietary energy to fuel the modern age.

The African kids would presumably benefit from some energy-rich, even if nutrient-poor, food like sugar. Vice versa, what a gene-poor Parisian needs is not to renounce their *madeleine* but to make sure they don't forget to give chicory to the madding crowd below.

While there are several efforts to classify a few general microbiome regimes, that may be just an heuristic as individual differences appear to be very marked and human environments can be vastly diverse. Examples of how it is hard to formulate general rules emerged clearly in studies of the Hazda, in Tanzania, that is widely seen as one of the most pristinely pre-industrial communities alive today. Enthusiasm about the so-called "Paleolithic diet" has spurred intense study of just who they keep as commensal guests. It turns out they have hardly any *Bifidobacteria,* which appeared to be highly beneficial in the Shanghai and many other experiments and is commonly added to probiotic health drinks. Their guts had high counts of *Treponema,* associated with irritable bowel syndrome and various other metabolic problems that, however, the Hazda do not experience.

Curiously, the Hazda microbiome was not only different from that found elsewhere but men and women had quite different intestinal populations. The differences suggest that women eat more fiber and men more meat and honey – reflecting the Hazda's cultural occupation patterns. So while hunters and gatherers may warrant acclaim as egalitarians, they must do a fair bit of snacking on the job. Indeed, Hazda people eat about a third of their food away from camp, about the same as Americans today.[42]

Lastly, while 90 percent of a typical Italian's diet comes from easily digestible starches and sugars – reflecting millennia of agriculture – the Hazda have virtually no farm food, and absolutely no dairy products, instead eating baobab, berries, and tubers along with meat and honey. Tubers are important – they represent a natural food storage system if you leave them in the ground – but even the Hazda don't particularly like them. They eat them raw or after a quick roast and actually spit out much of the tough fiber. While the very broad array of tubers eaten likely brings in a wide raft of micronutrients and fosters gut biodiversity, what the Hazda themselves actually ingest from them is roughly half simple sugars and another quarter starch – not at all what champions of the Paleolithic diet currently so much in vogue would advocate![43]

So how, if they eat sugar and simple carbohydrates, do they stay so thin?

Actually, they stay small, and don't have desk jobs. Much is made of how much they walk – 12 kilometers a day for men with their bows and arrows, six for women who however use digging sticks to forage. But in the end, adjusted for height and body weight – adjusting for a BMI typically around 20 – total Hazda energy expenditure isn't really any different than the typical western adult.[44]

Evidently the Hazda's foraging style brings in a broad diversity of foods and so they keep their gut guests in line. It likely helps that, while they do eat a lot of sugar, with daily intake of honey accounting for 15 percent of their annual calories, they do not accompany it with abundant fats and meats.

Interestingly, honey accounts at times for up to 80 percent of the diet of Mbuti Pygmies. A 23-man honey-hunting camp in eastern Zaire consumed 229 kilograms of honey in 12 days, translating to almost a kilogram per person per day. Mituso Ichikawa, the Japanese anthropologist accompanying them, estimated that after subtracting wax and adding in a bit of on-site snacking, each Mbuti took in 1,900 calories a day of honey. However, they don't even think about eating cheeseburgers during this brief seasonal splurge.

In a sign of sugar's importance to them, the surplus take is wrapped in leaves and distributed to other camp members as well as members of rival bands in coded gift exchanges. "Although they give honey to other persons with the expectation of its return they never do so based on the strict calculation of the amount given and taken," Ichikawa says, highlighting honey's key mediating role in Mbuti social metabolism.[45]

It turns out that honey, apart from being sweet and 90 percent sugar and water, also has an inhibitory impact on around sixty known bacterial species in the gut, which no doubt is why it is so often known as a medicinal food. Those attributes reflect components such as organic acids, which account for around 0.6 percent of honey and around 1 percent of mineral compounds, including potassium, magnesium, and phosphorous, as well as various vitamins, a set of relevant enzymes and a tiny amount of protein.[46]

All of these elements, such a tiny part of honey by volume, are of great interest to the microbiome. But the desire for honey, depicted countless times in archaeological relics and one of the catalysts for the hominid emergence from the primate pack, reflects a conscious desire for sugar, which provides energy for brains and bodies. Pure sucrose from refined sugar cane is, as noted, a turbocharged form of photosynthesis for humans rather than a complex deep-ecological ensemble. Indeed, its refinement to near perfect chemical purity strips it of those non-digestible prebiotic goodies stressed by Zhao. It's just an efficient energy source.

Maybe that's why people don't eat sugar with spoons. It accompanies other foods; except for candy, but nobody lives on candy alone, except perhaps for Andy Warhol. Remarkably, much of this was hinted at in a

1972 article in which a California laboratory that worked with cases of extreme obesity gave three healthy volunteers a chemically-pure synthetic diet based on glucose and found that they were able to survive quite well on very low calorie counts, suggesting a very efficient harvest of energy from the soluble powder. Bifidobacterium completely disappeared from their stool samples, while *Bacteroidetes* counts diminished.[47]

Their throwaway hunch was that colonic bacteria probably survived by chewing up old epithelial gut-wall cells. Today such an outcome would be read as a pathological reaction, interestingly based on the lack of phytochemicals and micronutrients arriving at the lower intestine because the chemical diet constituted, instead of sugar, fat, synthetic vitamins, and emulsifiers. That's a fiber-free formula the scientists thought might work during space travel.

While that hints at a brave new world where people eat hyper energy-efficient synthetic foods and become like germ-free mice, it also underscores that such a menu tends to trigger metabolic calamities as key gut microbes are not fed. It's not a matter of what's present but of what's missing.

The question is whether we can ever be the boss of our bacteria. On that note, there are a few bacterial species that Zhao and several other research teams have keyed in on as a possible magical anti-obesity machine: one is the *Akkermansia muciniphila*. This genus was identified in 2004 and appears to subside in obese microbiomes and thrive in lean ones. The species in question appears to increase the thickness of the epithelium wall – with mucus, hence its name – thus blocking the transfer of food to the blood supply. The thicker the gut wall, the less likely bacteria can trigger inflammation responses.

This species has also been found to be prevalent in the microbiomes of elite athletes, who tend to have high consumption of sugar, fat, and protein. A study of rugby players also found greater microbial diversity, which appears to be a sure plus.[48]

While studies of people show this species' inverse correlation with obesity, studies with mice have gone further, and shown that raising *Akkermansia muciniphila* counts can lead to weight loss and improved insulin resistance. Moreover, they do not require vast regime changes to prevail, so appear to be central actors on the metabolic scene.[49] What remains unclear is just how to make them bloom, but scientists and commercial laboratories are working hard on probiotic products designed to do just that, and some marketers have already rolled out items – such as organic psyllium seed husk – they say will at least maintain existing colonies of the bacteria. On the flip side, another species, *Methanobrevibacter smithii*, is poised to become a target for obliteration as it appears to be a ringleader in helping the lower intestine harvest more energy for its human host, which might be adaptive for those with high-fiber diets but is the opposite for those with access to highly palatable snack foods.

Despite the excitement about an imminent miracle cure leading to weight loss for all – just as a single drug was used to knock out polio for everyone – it's important to remember that the microbiome is itself an ecosystem and one existing in a network of many others. Species are not good or bad. This need not be a military campaign, and anyway achieving a consensus on the platonic form of the human microbiome would likely be a daunting task with unpredictable and probably unwelcome side effects. That jars a bit with the outward norms of the Anthropocene, the era when we humans call the shots.

At the same time, there is no reason to assume that efficiency rules in nature. Consider the giant panda. Sequencing of its gut microbiota confirmed that it really is a bear-like carnivore although it eats bamboo. In a way, the animal is not very clever; indeed, its brain and other organs are smaller than they should be. Pandas are incredibly slow and spend very little energy beyond their basal metabolism rate, which is comparable, when adjusting for size, to that of a lizard. Giant pandas eat bamboo. It turns out they lost a taste-controlling gene that drove them to eat meat but don't have enough cellulose-digesting enzymes to crack their preferred dietary fiber and so they spend 14 hours a day eating up to a third of their body weight in stalks and shoots.[50]

Pandas have a strong sweet tooth. One of the ironies of their choice of bamboo, a C4 plant, is that they can't digest 80 percent of what they eat. In short, they eat far too many fibers and are on a calorie-restricted diet. They're close to a state of torpor, and yet they have for two million years coped with a low-diversity, obesogenic microbiome. They persevere. They are doing what we may one day be forced to do: self-evolve our metagenomics superorganism. It's a slow and not very exciting destiny, perhaps even one it's best to avoid.[51] But the panda shows it can be done. The animal is "aberrant and enigmatic," but that's part of the reason it is a Chinese national treasure, says Zhengsheng Xue, a colleague of Zhao in Shanghai.

Resilience and Rapidification

6

There is something that causes me the greatest difficulty, and continues to do so without relief: unspeakably more depends on what things are called than on what they are.

Friedrich Nietzsche[1]

Richard Oster, a medical researcher at the University of Alberta, has noticed a quirk in how health problems are propagating across Canada's First Nations populations. Indigenous peoples around the world have some of the highest obesity and diabetes rates ever recorded, attributed to newly sedentary lifestyles and the kind of refined-carbohydrate-and-fat diet known as western chow. Prevalence of diabetes ranges as high as 18 percent in some Canadian groups, five times higher than those in the rest of the national population, fitting neatly into a long-established pattern that is also eminently visible among Native Americans and Australian Aborigines.

After years of observation Oster was happy to note a deceleration in the growth of diabetes among First Nations in his province, although he was troubled that it remained high. Then he shifted his routine data-crunching methods and, with the collaboration of local Cree and Blackfoot community leaders, pursued a more granular approach. He found that groups with high knowledge of their native language had sharply lower diabetes rates than those without – by a factor of three overall, and up to 15 for some communities. Those are adjusted findings, meaning they stand after income, smoking, and other lifestyle or contingent factors have been factored out. They suggest that people with high "cultural continuity" have fewer eating disorders. No wonder wedding parties tend to be so big and fat! That those First Nations communities which have managed to preserve their culture – language being the proxy – appear to benefit from protection from diabetes and obesity is extraordinary in many ways.

In the hundreds of interviews about diabetes and health issues done for the research, Oster and his colleagues constantly heard people refer to the importance of "being who we are" and emphasize that loss of culture leads to a state of woe. Everyone recognizes that the days of trapping and living off the land are gone, but for some reason more than 90 percent of the members of some communities speak their native tongue, while only one in ten of other groups do.[2]

Oster told me he doesn't think that western chow has no role in the higher-than-average health woes of Alberta's indigenous people – poverty and a poor diet often go together – but that using such a narrow lifestyle paradigm was very short-sighted and unnecessarily superficial, especially for a problem that is proving elusive for Canada's substantial public health and welfare systems. "Many of these people live in a constant state of crisis and grief, so lifestyle falls pretty low on the list of priorities," he said, noting that cultural resilience can not only provide stability during turbulent times but can also "lead to less chronic stress, which itself has been linked to the development of diabetes. So not everything goes through the lifestyle channel."

Canada's indigenous peoples were definitely facing extreme and lasting stress in the middle of the twentieth century, as the fur trade collapsed around the 1920s, leading many households to live on calorie counts below those later used in Ancel Keys' famous starvation experiment using conscientious objectors in Minnesota. Indeed, nutrition authorities essentially conducted a series of extreme randomized controlled trials on children forced to attend residential schools, as many as half of whom died. These continued until the 1950s.[3] The root causes of most of the health problems that First Nations populations disproportionately suffer from stem from colonialism, Oster said.[4]

This is a common complaint but it is not some political wailing or a new-age dogma. It is a striking plain-vanilla epidemiological correlation – perhaps not as strong as a genetically obese rat's developing diabetes on a 70 percent fructose diet, but numerically more robust than the countless studies on sugary beverages. If removing barriers to cultural continuity reduces diabetes prevalence by a factor of three, it may offer clues as to how to obtain far more bang for the health care buck than reimbursing weight-loss drugs, banning soda from shops, or endorsing implausibly low sugar quotas.[5]

Culture, a legacy not a conundrum

Addressing culture's role in human affairs inevitably ends up leading to a brambly thicket, but the same is true of today's canonical view that non-communicative diseases are the products of "lifestyle" flaws and as such can be reversed with specific behavioral changes. We are already neck-deep in the bog. This point was taken up poignantly by Richard Eckersley of Australian National University when he floated the idea that, as regards metabolic diseases, modern western culture itself is the risk factor par excellence. While his definition of the culprit is a value system dominated by materialism and individualism, he cogently notes that he is referring to culture not just as a demarcation between social groups but rather as an inclusive generator of an array of instinctive behavioral codes, conveyed as whispered suggestions rather than shouted out as commands. Exonerating individualism as a progressive force in history, he proposes that materialism, through the stress of the acquisitive drive and its mediation through high requisite self-esteem, actually lowers standards of living for most of those who aspire to its rewards.[6]

While commendable for trying to put meat on the bones of the culture concept so frequently cited and then forgotten in the opening preambles to public-health research papers, Eckersley perhaps overlooks the fact that life is not stress-free outside of western culture. Many animals are maniacally status-oriented, and on the Melanesian island of Kitava, touted for its inhabitants' practically sugar-free diet and superb cardiovascular health despite rampant tobacco smoking, one of the leading causes of death is suicide – usually by diving head first from a coconut tree – after a serious social gaffe or snub.

Evidence suggests that it is when cultures are disrupted, derailed, and decimated that troubles emerge, and often on a slow boil. It is deeply misleading to identify a culture with its shadowy bare survival, which is one reason why the idea of a "culture of poverty" failed to gain traction in the social sciences – even though it has stealthily entrenched itself into elite bureaucratic language, often with some perfunctory clause about the duty to respect all social traditions.[7]

Genetics and its corollary disciplines are increasingly finding culture to be a causal power, and there are biological pathways for the impact of unsolicited rapid cultural change, which after all is not an experience reserved for indigenous peoples in settler societies. Researchers have found that scores of genes express themselves differently in individuals who feel socially isolated as opposed to those who do not, and the bulk of these involve triggering inflammatory reactions. Likely a primordial way to upgrade defenses against infection after suffering a wound, these changes can be long-lasting, sometimes remaining in the personal programming of people born in poverty who manage to escape it – hinting at a physiological pathway for all the troubling correlations between social factors and metabolic disorders.

One key channel entails cortisol, a hormone the body releases in response to stress and which stimulates greater glucose production in a bid to restrain excess inflammation. This occurs through, and can lastingly influence, the workings of the HPA or hypothalamic-pituitary-adrenal axis, one of the main links between our brain and our endocrinal system. As such it is quite likely a pathogenic mechanism in the genesis of diabetes and obesity.

Here's how it works. The hypothalamus issues extra cortisol in situations of stress, the cause of which can range from an unexpected barking dog, a physical injury or loneliness to marital wobbles, a menacing memo from your employer's human resources department, or living in an overcrowded apartment in a dangerous neighborhood. Cortisol is an alarm bell which puts your body on alert, blocking extraneous activities such as digestion and immunological maintenance to focus on a fight-or-flight decision – which can sometimes play out as a hide-or-freeze choice.

These moments can be existentially decisive for prey animals, so the body has an app for that. When the dog stops barking, or the challenge passes, the cortisol drops and things go to back to normal. But many Anthropocene stresses persist. Laboratory rats in cages, for example, remain in agitation for up to ten days after seeing a cat. And a new study of healthy Italians found that stresses related to low socioeconomic status trigger lesser DNA methylation of genes meant to govern the immune system, suggesting that chronic disease risk can take the form of biological software in real time.

Because cortisol – which is abundant in people with Prader-Willi Syndrome, the genetic obesity condition – counteracts insulin and regulates adipose tissue, its extended circulation can initially lead to slimming, but after a while visceral obesity begins, and if chronic or repetitive stress exhausts the HPA's regulatory mechanisms, cortisol levels collapse and metabolic syndrome sets in.[8]

This kind of stress has been empirically associated with people in situations of subordination – which as the Whitehall study of London's civil servants points out is distinct from being poor – and has been widely observed at work on animals. Even wild animals have the reaction, be it to food scarcity or an unusually high presence of predators. Up to a point it's adaptive, as when a rabbit sees a fox it really shouldn't dawdle to nab one last bit of dietary fiber. Among primates, where status hierarchies are frequent, cortisol may surge in a challenge situation, and persist in a low-level way for the loser, leading to forms of behavior such as withdrawal, resignation, and obsessive off-hours snacking.

Such defeat can have quite shocking outcomes among rats. A famous experiment half a century ago found that victorious alpha rats would engage in rape, pillage, and infanticide while, stressed-out mothers stopped making nests and abandoned their children and loser males split between aggressive sexual deviancy or living like zombies, eating their ad libitum pellets while ignoring and being ignored by the others.[9]

Contemporary understanding of the HPA mechanism has allowed for stress to be understood not only as a reaction to an event but also as the anticipation of potential trouble.

Syrian hamsters, typically solitary and highly territorial, reacted to crowded cages by becoming overweight even though they didn't eat more, as their HPA command center instructed them to keep calm and thus channeled more dietary energy into adipose tissue. And while the males of many naturally communitarian rodent species tend to establish stable hierarchies fairly quickly, with low-status individuals doomed to lose weight – they shed lean tissue not fat cells – the reaction is different when they are subjected to the repeated entry into their cage of an intruder. Filled with a sense of worry and dread, the loser will start to develop metabolic syndrome and become obese. The response is seen as an advantageous survival strategy but if prolonged becomes slowly lethal as chronic stress erodes the machinery of the HPA signaling pathway, eroding insulin sensitivity and even blunting satiety.

These metabolic consequences derive from social conflict alone. One test found that both dominant and subordinate mice forced to engage in conflict were happy to over consume a high-fat diet, but only the latter became diabetic and obese, while the former appeared to prefer a sugar-rich carbohydrate diet they could turn into fuel.[10]

While stressed individuals – rodents and humans alike – do appear to develop a hankering for fatty or sweet "comfort foods", it is not clear that the dietary channel is needed as a path to obesity, as chronic stress appears to redesign the endocrinological workings and metabolic allocations independently of food, even creating a new phenotype predisposed to weight gain. And, since cortisol's most conspicuous effect involves regulating metabolism and raising energy demands, it is worth noting that it triples among chimpanzees when ripe figs are out of season, depriving them of their main source of simple sugars![11]

The irony is that the HPA axis, in releasing cortisol in response to stress, is signaling that it will tap all available energy. So when rodents in cages, or people, realize it's a false alarm, they orient to sugar-stuffed cookies and hyper-palatable foods, which attenuate the alarm. The system works, but at cross purposes if the adverse conditions last too long.[12]

Sound familiar?

In making the leap to humans, one question might be to wonder how today's leaders, thriving in a competitive and meritocratic society, manage to control their legendary stressful lives. But the stress referred to here is not folklore but biological, linked to fight-or-flight responses and measurable initially by cortisol levels. High-ranked business and military leaders tend in fact to have lower cortisol levels, suggesting that leadership itself helps keep a metabolic house in order.[13]

Low homeostatic cortisol levels also appear to allow for sharper reactions to acute stress, allowing for superior performance in fight-and-flight situations as well as quicker healing times from injury and illness. This shows that some stress is beneficial, as it exercises the body's in-house self-protection systems, for which after all the HPA-mediated flight-or-fight response has evolved. But it all backfires if stress is chronic.

Alpha leaders of a gang of status-conscious wild baboons could in practice actively exploit such differentiated responses as a weapon to maintain dominance over their ever-weakening rivals. So the beatings and chase scenes, often involving screaming, seen among primate groups in the wild are indeed political.[14]

Among more egalitarian animals, cortisol surges occur frequently, explaining the anarchic fighting between African wild dogs, or spotted hyenas when on the open savannah. Dominant primates also sometimes endure cortisol surges themselves – almost always at revolutionary times when an alpha figure faces an explicit challenge to its supremacy.[15]

That might explain why diabetes emerged and was considered a disease of affluence when it cropped up in the late 1600s, in the 1800s, and again in the 1920s – all times when rapid social change led to rearranged power relations and existing elites faced heightened stress as new breeds of industrialists staged their successful campaign to replace rentiers atop the social order. The relative lack of mobility in advanced nations may help explain the rarity of obesity among today's elite, while the opposite dynamic explains growing obesity rates among the higher-echelon of developing countries.

Of course, caution is required when assessing the relevance to humans of what animals do, notes Robert Sapolsky, professor of biology and neuroscience at Stanford University and a leading expert on the role of environmental stress on cortisol secretion. Caution is especially in order with animals in captivity or in laboratory cages, as they endure the anomaly of being unable to avoid dominant individuals even if they wish it. The zombie mice referred to earlier would presumably have abandoned their endless supply of sweetened chow pellets and pushed off for a more austere habitat if they had been free to leave their dystopia.

Moreover, a casual temptation to associate low status with low socioeconomic position may miss the point that stress-induced changes are biological, involving a reworked "neurochemistry of anxiety" replete with apposite synthetic molecules. That doesn't mean there isn't a connection, though, only that diseases like diabetes shouldn't be linked to something like limited access to public health care. The stress connection is far deeper and more mechanical than lifestyle differences such as smoking, drinking, exercise, or current diet. Insofar as our individual selves are concerned, according to Sapolsky, the adverse stress mechanism is rather subjective and even consists of "being made to feel poor by one's surroundings."[16] That subjectivity and relativism is borne out repeatedly in relatively comfortable economic situations. For example, boredom and anomie, in the sense of doing something that makes little sense, is another diabetic predictor, according to an interesting study of 5,000 Swedish working women. Maybe Marabou chocolates or dill-flavored chips were hidden in their desk drawers, but those whose jobs gave them a low "sense of coherence" were more at risk of diabetes than those with routine or highly demanding but satisfying jobs. Interestingly, jobs with a low decision latitude but a high sense of coherence also had no association with greater risk.[17]

Justice also gets its due. Male London civil servants who felt that workloads were not equitably distributed and that promotions were not guided by merit ended up with a 25 percent higher chance of developing metabolic syndrome, and a 33 percent higher chance of becoming obese, according to the Whitehall study.[18] That suggests that fairness shortfalls, even in the ostensibly rule-governed modern bureaucratic workplace, are part of the social stress gradient by which diabetes is spread – in fact they pose an extra risk similar to more than two extra sodas a day!

More importantly, this brings us back to what Oster discovered. Indigenous communities able to maintain cultural resilience have far less prevalence of diabetes than those that for whatever reasons were unable to do so. Evidence abounds of that pattern from the Caribbean to Samoa. Among the Tsimane of Amazonian Bolivia, cardiovascular health is highest, and cortisol lowest, among those with the most cultural clout, meaning that there still is some. Clout reflects prestige, not dominance, and is obtained by credible mediation skills, not money. To be sure, the Tsimane buy in only 10 percent of their food, leaving them relatively autarkic and making face-to-face cultural interactions still the salient channel. In fact, cortisol and blood pressure are highest among Tsimane with the greatest cash income, who are likely frustrated at how poor they remain compared to the local townsfolk even while at home they are considered less adept at traditional skills such as hunting.[19]

Of course, there often comes a time when the colonial settler arrives, the urban ring road cuts through the family farm, one packs up and moves to the big city, when the village-style paradigm gives way to the prevalent urban, globalizing one. Such lurching changes, which almost always include new food supplies, are themselves harbingers of metabolic woes. One can only hope they are also the beginning of a transition to a new equilibrium.

Some say agriculture itself, with its exploitation of simpler carbohydrates, marked such an epochal transition and entailed a human health calamity greater even than the uprooting of rural peasants at the time of London's "gin epidemic." Much of modernity may be indigestible. Perhaps we should forget engineered palatability; it's time to order sugar and salt-free pizzas made with hand-ground acorn flour, topped with freshly-ripened tomatoes and slabs of winter bison meat, and sprinkled with just-in-time wild asparagus shoots.

For those caught on the back foot – whose culture or socioeconomic position was denied or lost resilience – the phenotypic rift is dramatic. An idea that's not for this book is that we ourselves are being domesticated and are unconsciously using stress, diet, grouchy microbes, and epigenetic changes to fashion a wholly new genome. Scientists who recently cracked the secret of the recent domestication of the rabbit – a prey animal primed for flight – describe its genetic transformation as a process much like diabetes, which has many shapes and causes and amounts to an adaptation run amok.[20]

As for cats and dogs, well, they were domesticated much earlier – and it turns out that more than half of them are already overweight or obese.[21]

Inheriting a metabolic ghetto

Apart from the prospects for devising stress-reduction therapies to coax bodies out of their pre-programmed funk, or of developing drugs that do the same job directly, there is an open question of whether these epigenetic changes can be inherited. Several laboratory studies suggest that stress as an infant – such as early separation from a mother – can crop up as depression when the mouse is ready to reproduce. Assessing such hereditability among people is harder due to the myriad factors that presumably characterize the life of someone who, for example, was born to the survivor of a genocide or concentration camp but now lives amid seeming plenty.[22]

It may seem we have traveled far from sugar, but by digging deeper into what we think of as individual responses to cultural shock we have moved very close to the causal dynamics of the primary demonic health problems it is alleged to cause.

At any rate, the dietary link might be restored by junk foods – those fiber-free and palatable things we eat when blue or in need of solace from whatever life has thrown our way and it is all about us. But ignoring the cause of woe – which may ultimately date back to long ago – and simply taking these comfort foods away would likely constitute a further "insult" – the marvelous term physiological researchers use to describe a malnutrition shock.[23] The greatest insult was colonialism, which did not happen so long ago. In fact, as laboratory-rat studies are showing epigenetic transfers have spanned a dozen generations, its heyday was quite recent.

And today, 70 years after independence, India is the world leader in diabetes prevalence. While much work is being done on contemporary malnutrition in South Asia, Jonathan Wells, a nutrition expert at University College London, takes the long view of what he calls "maternal somatic capital," an asset that is acquired or lost across generations. There can be cases of rapid and drastic depredation of such capital, as occurred during the Dutch "hunger winter" of 1944, when drastic ration cuts – down to as few as 400 calories a day – were imposed by occupying German forces. Children born or conceived during this five-month period of near starvation have gone on to develop obesity, insulin resistance, and diabetes at unusually high rates in their 50s and 60s, which is widely seen as evidence that infants are imprinted by the conditions of their birth and may suffer overload as they later catch up and enter a normal and prosperous dietary environment. Similarly, a new and large-scale study of 325,000 Austrians now receiving pharmaceutical treatment for diabetes found a "massive excess risk" of incurring the disease among people born during and immediately after the country's three major famines, in 1918, 1938, and the two years after World War II ended. In what is by far the most quantitatively intense demographic analysis, it turns out that a famine-borne child had a 42 percent higher risk of becoming diabetic as an adult.[24]

Many peoples, especially under colonialism but also later as migrants, have endured somewhat milder privations but spread over multiple generations. Wells describes this as tantamount to a "metabolic ghetto," exit from which is much trickier than simply following contemporary nutrition guidelines. As he puts it, "public health policies need to benefit metabolic capacity without exacerbating metabolic load." What this means is that the regulatory organs such as the heart, liver, kidneys, and pancreas of a child born to maternal somatic poverty may need to grow in a controlled way, avoiding rapid normalization. Sadly, that may mean skipping dessert.

Call it the Leningrad solution. Children born during the siege of that city, which lasted five times longer than the Dutch hunger winter, also faced fetal and infant malnutrition but later obesity outcomes were less of a problem as they did not go on to enjoy supermarkets with more than 100 breakfast cereal brands.

The metabolic ghetto is the bitter fruit of an epigenetic process, replete with DNA methylation, and perhaps the only ideal way to avoid it is to make sure one's grandmother had a strong nutritional balance sheet herself. Some components function as liquid capital, meaning they can be acquired or lost quickly, as is the case for vitamins or energy stores. But others are illiquid capital and mature over much longer time frames – the mother's own stature, for example, or her level of lean tissue. Ultimately, intangibles and externals such as education or a refrigerator can also be incorporated into this elegant balance-sheet model, which adds family, culture, and history to the food pyramid.

The ultimate health-determining formula is the rate of maternal investment in the baby, which in turn hangs on the mother's current seasonal energy needs, her status regarding access to liquid resources, and her patrimony, whose depreciation can and must be managed. The beauty of this system is that mammals are designed to buffer contingent situations in the interest of their offspring and species. However, prolonged privations are an ecological emergency and the opposite occurs as capital is depleted.[25]

Many imperial subjects, Wells notes, endured the latter situation for a long time, creating a metabolic ghetto marked by lower stature, a measure he sees as a more subtle and sophisticated indicator of real population well-being than brute and easy-to-manipulate economic proxies such as gross domestic product. What's remarkable about India is that average stature continued to decline until the mid-twentieth century, long after European peoples began their rebound from the trials of the enclosure movement and the poorhouse. Indians lost their somatic capital over time, and liquid capital was also hard to obtain as colonial ships took local crops elsewhere.

What this translates to is that Indian children, especially girls, are often low birth weight but what they are missing is lean mass rather than adiposity. The "thin-fat child" is basically geared up to seek liquid capital – energy, carbohydrates – rather than rebuild somatic capital. That explains why one Indian agronomist, writing about sugar cane cultivation, described sugar and the local *jaggery* drink as "an effective remedy for thinness"![26]

Wells notes that the newborn body's focus on fat here is a good risk-management strategy for survival in harsh conditions but that it comes at the cost of perpetuating low metabolic capacity – which becomes a special liability today when many Indians are migrating to cities, whether it be to enjoy new prosperity or to be obliged to consume the cheapest foods available.[27]

Today, diabetes rates are amply into the double-digit territory in Indian cities, peaking at one in six in Hyderabad, and it occurs frequently at low BMI and sugar consumption rates by global standards.[28]

A theater near you

Thinking about metabolic diseases as the expression of events from long ago casts the foodie mantra of "eat only what your grandmother would have eaten" in a new light and offers insight into how the epidemic travels.

Consider the Pima Indians of southern Arizona, who once ate more legumes than anyone on earth but for decades have been studied as the population with the highest rate of diabetes in the world – now around 40 percent – and nearly universal obesity for decades. Scientists have ransacked the Pima genome for signs of susceptibility, but finding none – their brethren in Mexico seem to be doing fine – the consensus is that their illness reflects their modern diet of refined ground flour, sugar, low-protein pinto beans, bacon lard, and sweetcorn. The component of fats in their overall diet has tripled.[29]

But what is often neglected is that the Pima, who integrated Spanish wheat, melons, and cattle into their farms centuries ago and regularly supplied food to passing wagon trains in the 1800s, suffered from starvation in the late nineteenth century, due to a drought lasting more than a decade exacerbated by the diversion of their Gila River water resources.[30] They have never recovered their prosperity nor their water but they did – like many other Native American groups, routinely described as in excellent physical condition before being harried and marched to reservations – eventually receive government food rations, essentially giving them liquid capital but depriving them both culturally and economically of access to somatic capital.

Extreme food insecurity probably lasted for 70 years, according to Daniel Benyshek, an anthropologist who has worked extensively with

Arizona tribal communities. "Diabetes is a political disease" and initial genetic theories often rapidly degenerate into the pretext for reprimanding people for their lifestyles, he says.[31]

In a clockwork example of the metabolic ghetto at work through fetal malnutrition followed by frybread – a palatable use of the lard, flour, and sugar they were given as rations – two generations later diabetes afflicted half of Pima adults, and yet another two generations later most children are born to diabetic mothers.[32]

Variants of the same storyline apply to Australia's Aboriginals. Anecdotal evidence suggests that some individual Aboriginals and Pima have mitigated or even reversed their diabetic state by reverting to traditional hunting-and-gathering lifestyles, which while certainly a decision with dietary significance is also a supremely political gesture whose viability on a large scale would probably require reinventing cultural capital and would obviously stoke conflict over land ownership.

A further and perhaps unexpected version of the metabolic ghetto – and possibly the indicator of an eventual escape route – comes in the relation between Jewish peoples and diabetes. Jews in the late nineteenth and early twentieth century, especially in cities like Vienna, Berlin, and Boston, were depicted as particularly susceptible to the disease, which in German even came to be known as *Judenkrankheit*.[33]

Stereotyping is part of culture and so interesting itself, especially as the association of diabetes with Jews rapidly disappeared in the 1930s, more or less simultaneously with the recognition the disease was growing fast among black Americans. What is intriguing, though, is that late nineteenth-century accounts in Europe regularly described the growing number of urban Jews as short in stature – a sign that perhaps they were recovering from a previous period of malnutrition in Eastern European *shtetls*, where dietary intakes had recently fallen below 2,000 calories, most of them from bread. The steady collapse of regional peasant economies in the 1800s triggered large-scale migration to cities, where food supplies were steadier.

Diet and nutrition were a mixed picture in the U.S. at the time. On the one hand, in the prosperous urban northeast, Americans were famously big eaters on the caloric front, although nutritional balances were subprime as the menu was heavy on carbohydrates and slabs of meat, both of which were deemed easier to digest.

The table below shows some of Wilbur Olin Atwater's dietary estimates from 1894.

The carbohydrate measure is by weight, in pounds. The fuel value is measured in kilocalories, and the nutritive value is the ratio of protein to the sum of fat and carbohydrates. Protein intake varied from 18 pounds for a Munich lawyer to two and a half times as much for a "hard-working" Lowell blacksmith. Fat intake ranged by a factor of nine between German peacetime army rations and Massachussetts brickmakers. Atwater attributed the high energy intake of the American working class to the fact that they "do more work than in Europe" but was perplexed why this would be true of the professional classes as well. The high nutritive ratio of Americans was not optimal, reflecting more meat-and-potatoes and less lean meat, fish, and beans, prompting him to observe that Americans eat too much fat, starch, and sugar. That, he said, reflected general ignorance about the uses and values of food. In his 1894 government publication, *Foods: Nutritive Value and Cost*, Atwater advocated a low-cost diet, noting that with 25 cents at a time one could purchase one pound of sirloin, 4.17 pounds of beef neck, 5 pounds of sugar or 20 pounds of potatoes.

A continental divide in work, energy and food costs

Who	Carbohydrates (lbs)	Fuel Value (kcals)	Nutritive ratio
Carpenter, USA	0.76	3,055	5.5
Blacksmith. USA	1.75	6,905	7.4
Brickmaker, USA	2.54	8,850	11
College student, USA	1.08	3,925	6.6
Blacksmith, England	1.47	4,115	4.8
Miners, Germany	1.40	4,195	6.7
German peacetime army ration	1.06	2,800	5
German wartime army ration	1.49	3,985	4.1
Lawyer, Germany	0.49	2,400	6.3
Italian brickmakers in Germany	1.49	4,540	5.6

But when the government conducted a set of house-to-house surveys in the late 1890s to collect information on what poor and minority households were eating, the accounts were sobering. Sacks of sugar outnumbered vegetable sightings, and it wasn't much of a match. Inspectors found malnutrition in 60 percent of the white households visited in Crooked Creek, an Appalachian hideaway. Southern comfort food still awaited its ingredients. Tenant farmers in Alabama had less than a fifth of the food diversity enjoyed by poor blacks in Philadelphia. Calorie intakes plummeted in the winter for everyone but urban professionals. Italians in Chicago wouldn't even let the researchers in the door. They were suspicious the real agenda was "to see how cheaply people could live so employers could cut wages accordingly."[34]

Exploring the ghetto

Is there any cultural evidence of metabolic ghettos formed in recent decades that might be fostering obesity by creating human phenotypes geared to liquid rather than somatic capital? And might there be some programmed high-cortisol "lifestyles" out there, braced in a fight-or-flight mode from childhood on and disposed to HPA burnout at age 50 or 60?

Genomic transcriptional profiling of a group of 103 healthy and moderately affluent 30-year-old Americans detected precisely that among those who had grown up in adversity, and that "biological residue" persisted independently of its carriers' lifestyle or even perceived stress.[35]

Meanwhile, a street-by-street analysis of Manhattan found a clear correlation of community-wide stress and BMI, with alarming diabesity prevalence tending to concentrate near the shatter zone where the city shifts from affluence to poverty right above Central Park. Another study of down-at-the-heel parts of St. Louis went even deeper and found that living in poor housing units doubled susceptibility to diabetes and was far more important than a dilapidated neighborhood.[36]

Similar biomarkers have been seen emerging quickly among Kenyan and Tanzanian migrants heading from the countryside to the capital, and is beginning to be seen among rural migrants to cities in India, where diabetes has mostly been an affliction of wealthier burghers. Insulin resistance also rose among one of the most educated groups in the world, Chinese immigrants in Pennsylvania, due to cultural stress evidently linked to social acculturation. Despite the relative success of this immigrant group, they come from a country that endured severe famine in the early 1960s and today one in eight of those born in China but now in the USA are diabetic, twice the national rate and higher than Hispanics.[37]

The big leap in obesity and overweight in the USA, an interesting crucible due to its apparent affluence, melting-pot population, and particularly rich archival data, began in the 1960s and accelerated in the 1980s. That offers some time markers that correspond to a host of novelties ranging from food factors such as the growing use of chemicals and antibiotics in food production, more than 12,000 new food additives including high-fructose corn syrup, ketchup's apocryphal anointment as a school-lunch vegetable (actually relish was put on the list), the dawn of big-box retail stores, and the sharp uptick in eating outside of the home, to measurable economic facts such as real wage stagnation, the shift from industry to service-sectors jobs, increasing economic inequality at the household level and lately an evident spatial concentration of poverty described as the resurrection of fully-fledged slums.[38]

That's a lot of dietary and social change. Add in that the majority of students in public schools now qualify for lunch subsidies, meaning they are from low-income homes, and one might shiver at what future epidemiological cohort studies will find. The Department of Agriculture calculates that 49 million Americans do not enjoy basic food security, meaning they either reduce consumption or increase their reliance on cheap and monotonous staple foods. The ranks of those facing outright cuts to their food supply has doubled since 2000.

Low income is an obvious cause, but the government's surveys show that income shocks – as in temporary job loss or salary cuts – also play a role, as can volatile housing costs. Both have been in ample supply since the global financial crisis erupted, but in fact spending on food has been on a downward spiral for some time. From 2000 to 2007, median spending on food by US households declined by 6 percent compared to the inflation measure pegged to food and beverages, and by twice as much compared to the cost of the government's own Thrifty Food Plan, which is designed to calculate the need for a food stamp program! That median figure masks a broad range, with the decline in food spending by those in the second-lowest income quintile falling by three times as much.[39]

As was seen with the decision to use public resources to bail out mortgage lenders rather than foreclosed home owners in the recent US housing market debacle, political opinions on why income and spending fell are likely to vary. That was also the case during the "gin epidemic" in England, when Hogarth and Fielding found it perfectly normal that the height gap between the rich and poor was a whopping 22 centimeters at age 16. Poor English kids were the shortest in Europe, while the affluent ones were the tallest. This domestic metabolic ghetto took generations to resolve, which is one reason why both colonial dynamics and the British policy interventions are so closely studied.[40]

But political predilections aside, cost-benefit analyses survive, and the North American evidence points to food insecurity generating sharply higher health care costs.[41] And if malnutrition is a ticket to higher future risks of metabolic syndrome and cardiovascular diseases, the bill is ready to grow.[42]

The drop in spending could of course be celebrated as a sign that the poorest are imbibing less sugary drinks and eating fewer cakes, and that they will benefit from their austerity. After more than a decade of steady annual declines, soda consumption in the USA is at 1986 levels.[43]

But official data notes those are the cheapest calories and possibly the last to leave the table in times of difficulty, which suggests that our gut microbes are not having a good time.

The complex dietary fibers that make it to our microbiome, where they are fermented and digested in a way that can protect our gut wall and properly regulate food digestion, have basically gone missing in the mainstream American diet. Total carbohydrate consumption at the end of the twentieth century was around 500 grams, nearly identical with its level 100 years earlier, but the trend charts a broad U-shape as it fell by 25 percent through 1964 before climbing back up. The percentage of fiber among those carbohydrates, meanwhile, plummeted much faster – by nearly 40 percent – in a decline that took place almost entirely in the period from 1945 to 1964, and never recovered. The bulk of the fiber loss came from processing whole grains into white flour, which increases caloric density by 10 percent but strips away fiber by 80 percent.[44]

While HFCS consumption began to take off in the 1980s, it mostly substituted for sugar, whose total consumption was higher in the late 1930s than in 1980, by which time obesity was already soaring, punctually one generation after a microbiome regime change. Pediatric obesity's peak waited one more twenty-five-year generation. The incidence of diabetes rose modestly throughout the century and then began to rise in earnest in the late 1990s.

Lack of dietary micronutrients, not excess sugars, fats or oils, drive the diabesity problem. In the words of Anne-Thea McGill, an innovative nutrition thinker from New Zealand, "the 'empty' part of 'empty calories' does matter." Our greatest health risk is not excess energy but the lack of the micronutrients that our gut microbes know how to convert to make our cells efficient in their use of energy.[45] That's borne out again in South Asian children living in Britain, a group known for obesity and worryingly high rates of diabetes – five times the national average among adults – who actually consume about 15 percent less sugar than the island's indigenous white people. They do eat more calories – almost 100 more a day – but these come from extra starch, polyunsaturated fats, and protein.[46]

They are short of vitamins C and D and, despite taking in more total iron, are also short on the heme iron the body needs. This group of youth probably eats less beef, but the deficiencies are a tell-tale sign that they aren't keen on leafy green vegetables. That is a common theme for South Asian emigrants elsewhere, and at home in India, too, where fruit and vegetable consumption in some regions is only 15 percent of WHO's recommended levels.[47]

However, it's hard to judge. People born in a metabolic ghetto are programmed to procure energy. Others, nutritionally, can have their cake and even eat it, but to maintain their stature should feed some fibers to their microbiome.

Public Policy and the Ghetto

7

We have often referred to "the scientific method." We now find that through applying it, we have moved from medicine into the social field, and in so doing we have had to consider some of the fundamental issues of our times.

Rudolph Virchow[1]

So we're back to where nutrition discourse always goes: if you want dessert, eat your spinach first. But doing the right thing will require you to dedicate some time, however, and time nowadays is money. "Cakes, cupcakes and cookies" have tracked generic US inflation for the past three decades, while the cost of fresh fruit and vegetables has outpaced it by around 2 percent a year, a pattern that hasn't been interrupted, according to government figures. Some claim that doesn't adequately factor in quality improvements for fresh produce, but that is a recent trend and is mainly about packing – pre-cut and pre-washed broccoli spears – with no impact on nutrition.[2]

In essence, lower-income households are nudged along the phenotypic trajectory wherein they shore up their liquid capital by consumption of energy foods, as the somatic capital of more nutrient-dense items is beyond their purchasing power. That meshes with the long-running campaign of Adam Drewnowski, a Seattle-based professor of nutrition who bluntly states: "Obesity rates in the United States are a function of socioeconomic status." Noting how the blame game shifts targets roughly each decade, he offers a more parsimonious formula: obesity is related to low-cost foods, and refined grains, added sugars, and added fats are all cheap, highly palatable and convenient. It is "the low cost of dietary energy, rather than specific food" or any inherent metabolic effects that track population weight gain, he says.[3]

It's a brutally simple explanation that can shoulder the data without sailing into obscurity. From the early 1970s through 2000, the availability of mostly refined flour and cereal products for Americans rose 48 percent, that of added fats and oils by 38 percent, and caloric sweeteners – comprising falling cane and beet sugar and rising HFCS – by 20 percent. Vegetables were amply available but that really testifies to iceberg lettuce, canned tomatoes, and above all potatoes, in the form of fries or chips, which together amounted to half the total vegetable count and five times the amount of more expensive dark-green, leafy and deep-yellow vegetables. These, together with fruit, doubled in retail price over fifteen years while sugar and fat flatlined. Because food is always described as cheap in America, affluent consumers may not notice just how much more expensive fiber has become for those who live and shop elsewhere.

Looking for single causes has tended to produce repetitive correlation studies drawn on too large a scale. This approach, Drewnowski notes, misses some striking facts. For example, sugar consumption's putative correlation with obesity breaks down when gender or geographical demands are made on the data. Moreover, sweetener consumption is very high among adolescent males but drops dramatically after age 24, suggesting that temporary but intense energy inputs are sought during a phase of life when people are striking out on their own. Asking low-income youth in that age bracket to drink more water doesn't sound like an easy job. It "seems particularly callous," adds Drewnowski.

Considering prices in terms of actual purchasing power can help untangle some of the confounding factors in big-data studies. Price, not the product, is often the obesogenic factor in play, he says, noting that 100 percent fresh-squeezed branded orange juice costs seven times more than the leading cola brand at a major supermarket chain. Their sugar loads are about equal.

Food budgets are already very different in US households. The top 20 percent by income spent 2.6 percent of their money on food but that still amounted to 50 percent more than that spent by those in the lowest quintile, for whom two-thirds as many dollars represent 19 percent of their income.

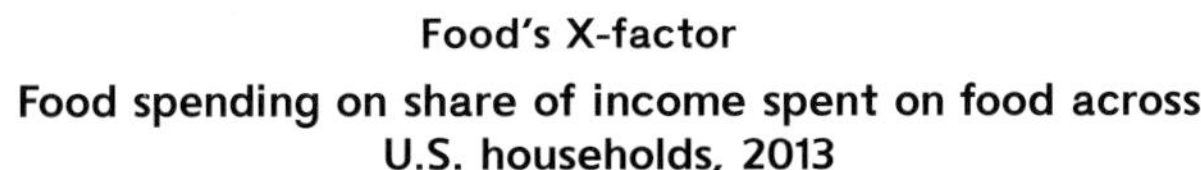

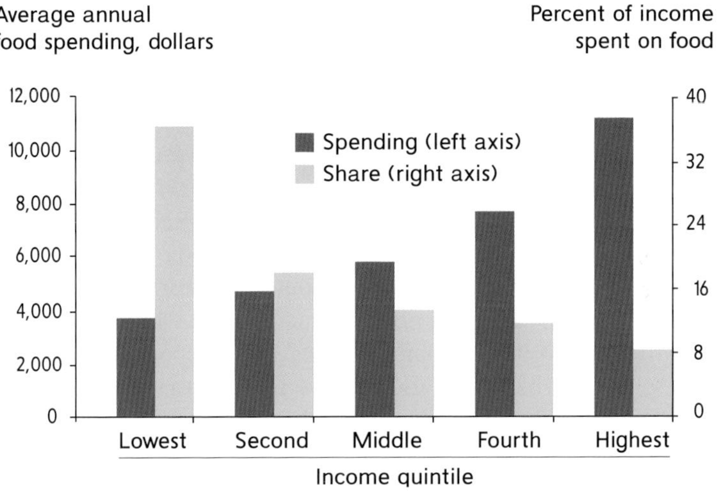

The graph tracks household food budgets in absolute dollar terms and as a share of income. An extra $100 a week for a three-person household would fund a nutrition transition to the Mediterranean diet. It would require a middle-class family to double its expenditure on food, while poorer households would be left with almost no income to spend on housing, clothing, education or any other needs

Source: US Department of Agriculture

Similar gaps exist in Europe and may even be larger in some cases, such as France, where four of every five households in the top quarter by income eat the recommended amount of fruit and vegetables compared to only one of every three of all the rest.[4] In Italy, where people enjoy making fun of American food habits, a leading newspaper exulted when local supermarket spending on fruit and vegetables overtook that on meat in the summer of 2015, celebrating it as a healthy turn and overlooking that it reflected higher prices for the former and benefited only exporters.

One study of a large group of well-educated Spaniards found that the typical cost of a Mediterranean diet – typically meaning high consumption of olive oil, vegetables, legumes, whole-grain products, fruits, and nuts with moderate amounts of fish and relatively little meat – is €1.35 more per day than a western diet for every 1,000 calories. That adds up to about $30 a week in extra costs per person, about equal to the entire current total outlay on food for a middle-class American family.[5]

The high salience of cost was recently highlighted in a sweeping cross-country way by the UK's Overseas Development Institute (ODI), which found that fresh green vegetable prices have been rising by 3.2 percent a year since 1990 in the UK, while snacks have been declining by around 0.3 percent. Since 1990, fresh produce prices have risen by up to 91 percent while processed ready-meals have dropped by up to 20 percent in emerging nations such as Brazil, China, Korea, and Mexico.[6]

The ODI report concludes that tax and subsidy interventions are required, but how to effect these without exacerbating the metabolic ghetto is not clear. Hiking the price of liquid capital while lowering it for long-term capital would, in financial terms, be a recipe for feudalism. The data presented in the report also offers a cornucopia of facts of interest to the dietary correlates to growing obesity. In urban China, for instance, vegetable prices are up by half since 1989 and sugar and rice are down by a quarter, but chicken is down by a third and oils are down by more than half. In Mexico, sugar prices are where they were in 1980 in inflation-adjusted real terms, while vegetable oils are lower by half.

That massive increase in the consumption of palm, soy, and other vegetable oils – all technically fats in the macronutrient framework – may have something to do with obesity and diabetes was even acknowledged recently by Barry Popkin, the scourge of sugar and dean of American dietary detectives. Urban Chinese may consume twice the recommended level of oils, and the country's imminent dietary health crisis will be bigger than America's, he recently told media in China, where he is leading a nutrition survey.[7]

An international team of scholars recently published a paper in the benchmark academic journal for obesity researchers that ought to have been candy for headline writers everywhere: "Vegetable-rich food pattern is related to obesity in China."

Due to the proliferating love of stir-fry methods since Beijing stopped its food rations system in 1988, vegetable consumption has become the vehicle for energy and is positively correlated with obesity! Remarkably, alternative dietaries – one described as "macho" and heavy on meat and alcohol, another dubbed "sweet tooth" and ample with cake, milk and

The changing American calorie map

Food type	1909	1999	Delta
Compositional changes in energy sources as a share of all calories			
Added sugars	10.64	16.95	+59%
Grains	36.75	22.43	–39%
Fruit, vegetables & legumes	9.85	8.4	–15%
Dairy	15.44	13.54	–12%
Meat including fish	13.65	14.93	+9%
Poultry	0.94	4.94	+526%
Oils, fats & shortening	11.25	19.82	+76%
Soybean oil	0.01	7.38	>738%
Shortening	2.17	5.67	+261%

The American dream of a chicken in every pot was largely realized in the twentieth century, as poultry consumption almost quintupled to 44 kilograms a person, a trend that began after 1945 when new techniques allowed the birds to grow faster and much larger. Sugar consumption grew inversely to grains, while total fats soared in the 1960s after doctors advised cutting back on animal fats. The shift in the type of fat tripled linoleic acid levels in adipose tissue and doubled it in breast milk. It also dramatically raised the ratio of n-6 to n-3 fatty acids, leading to reduced tissue concentrations of DHA and EPA, nutrients that act as anti-inflammatory agents as well as benefiting the gut's epithelial wall, fetal health, and the human retina. N-alpha-linolenic acids are typically found in fish, wild greens such as purslane, kiwi fruit, chia and flax seeds, cannabis, walnuts and, to a lesser extent, in olive oil. However, this type of n-3 PUFA oxidizes quickly, making it of less use in baking.

Source: Blasbalg T.L. *et al.*, "Changes in consumption of omega-3 and omega-6 fatty acids in the United States during the 20th century", *American Journal of Clinical Nutrition*, 2011, Vol. 93:5, pp. 950-962.

drinks – did not correlate with additional weight. There is actually no reason for that to sound crazy; it simply reflects the energy balance as followers of this diet consumed sugar without overdoing total calories, demonstrating that it's at any rate possible to do so.

The Chinese study is also interesting as it highlights cultural differences; western nutritionists have for centuries been unable to finish a sentence without praising vegetables, but in China eating them raw is not common and they are seen culturally as energy foods – because of the way they are actually consumed. A further wondrous example of a nutritional paradox is the fact that it is children of highly-educated Chinese families who say they engage in a lot of sports activities, eat plenty

Tracking the change

	1970	2010	Delta
China			
Total vegetable oils	4.74	21.05	344%
Of which, palm oil	0.37	5.44	1370%
Animal fats	10.16	52.71	419%
Of which, pork	7.83	35.41	352%
Total fats	14.90	73.76	395%
Total sugar	5.84	14.97	156%
Greece			
Total animal fats	29.22	43.22	48%
Of which, pork	2.19	10.48	379%
All oils	54.19	62.44	15%
Other than olive oil	1.95	21.66	1011%
Sugar	207	239	15%
Brazil			
Palm and soybean oil	4.84	42.28	774%
Sugar	98.45	100.05	2%
USA			
Total sweeteners	144.15	154.96	7%
Of which, sugar	121.46	73.33	-40%

Growing fat consumption, especially from vegetable oils, is by far the biggest dietary change in most of the world since 1970, besieging even countries once associated with the Mediterranean diet. (All measures in the table below are grams of fat per person per day. Sugar is measured in grams per person per day.)

For the record, in Italy, olive oil held steady, providing 30 grams of person per day throughout the period. Fat from soybean oil, cheese and pork grew from 20 grams to 51 grams

Source: FAOStat food balance sheets from UN Food and Agriculture Organization

of vegetables, and avoid sweets and fast-food restaurants who are the ones, it turns out from a study of 14,000 of them, who are most likely to be already overweight![8]

Let me learn to do it on my own

Food concepts do not easily cross borders due to cultural usages, nor are they so stable at home given that the affluent and the poor have remarkably little direct knowledge of what each other eat, nor what it costs or even tastes like. For example, Europe's posh like candy and pastries, whereas the rest eat cakes and are more likely to have table sugar at home. The French, meanwhile, have shifted to leaner meats across the board, a suggestive display of obedience to official advice.

Also striking is that while working-class Europeans enjoy saying that fresh produce is the healthy way to go, most have no intention of eating any themselves. Fruit and vegetables remain mainly on the plates only of elites, who in turn actually consider variety as the dietary high road. The poor, as it happens, are suspected of having meager cooking skills yet it is the rich who are most likely to eat convenience and ready-made foods. On that note, it may surprise some that low-income American households consume less sugar and HFCS than the national average.[9]

Despite the vast crunching of data – most of it collected via surveys relying on people to report what they eat without exaggerating – it seems we are grasping at straws. Experts tasked with drafting new dietary recommendations for Britain found that self-reported energy intake is 35 percent lower on average than total energy expenditure. The population should therefore be very slim and mostly dead![10] This, suggests Drewnowski, means public health proposals regarding nutrition will prove quite ineffective in reaching people who for whatever reason – cultural decimation, poverty, stress, indifference – are its elusive targets.

"The problem," Morten Larsen explained to me regarding the role of cheaper and processed energy-dense foods, "is that even if 'native' diets are better for everyone's health, they are not eaten for a multitude of social mechanisms and cultural reasons that might not have much to do with food specifically." Even if there were certainty over what the right diet is, "the question still remains as how to get people to eat it."

Larsen comes at the subject not as a nutritionist but as an expert in planning and development, teaching at Aalborg University in Denmark.

His Orwellian nightmare is that the nutrition elite will continue to search for the ideal diet while forgetting the particular situations of its proposed eaters. Assuming people are equally enabled rational individual consumers with similar food cultures and nutritional needs – of which they are probably unaware – is radically desocialized and part of a worrying trend to depoliticize expertise, he says.

George Orwell himself did some nutritional research when he explored the working-class peoples of Wigan Pier, an industrial zone near Manchester which had lost its canal-side pier long before the author visited in the late 1930s. One thing he quickly noted: "The peculiar evil is this, that the less money you have, the less inclined you feel to spend it on wholesome food." He wrote that in a milieu where urban pundits regularly deplored the horrors of what the lower classes ate – white bread, margarine, potatoes, tinned beef, and lots and lots of sugar in tea – and offered free advice on how to improve it, a behavior Orwell described as "cheeky" and compared to a high-society lady entering a slum home to "give shopping lessons to the wives of the unemployed." Interestingly, the Wigan Pier chow consisted almost exclusively of items previously introduced and recommended as safe by authorities exasperated by the spate of adulterated foods sold in the nineteenth century, mostly to working-class households who did not have a country manor or access to wholesome rural foods.

Larsen notes that a group of elite Scandinavian chefs and dieticians invented the "New Nordic Diet" in hopes of reviving local traditions. The dishes take quite a bit of time to prepare, which didn't help its reception beyond the already-affluent households who were keen to buy into the whole cultural package anyway. Those with more unstable economic foundations, especially if that status persists over generations, are likely to be cautious about change in general, even if what is held as traditional is itself quite new. For those who have no real reason to assume their lives are about to prosper, energy foods may be preferable as a way to cope with the stress of boredom. Moreover, Larsen notes, working-class people are likely to perceive outsiders' claims that they should adopt more "natural" habits as demeaning, and quickly dismiss them as ideological froth if the proposals are impractical and ignore their actual circumstances.

This was borne out in the almost surreally bold venture by Frances Hardin-Fanning, a professor of nursing at the University of Kentucky, when she sought to introduce the Mediterranean diet to Appalachia. She chose Breathitt County, an overwhelmingly white and English-speaking rural district where household incomes and university degrees are half the state average and a third of the population is classified as living in poverty. Some 47 percent are obese by the BMI metric and one in seven has been diagnosed with diabetes. That the county has only two grocery stores, both in the county seat, which is a 100-mile round-trip for a chunk of the population in the rugged former coal-mining area, added to the challenge.

Hardin-Fanning reached out to influential pastors in the county, a former moonshine and maple sugar center where the sale of alcohol is now illegal and most farms were sold to make way for the coal industry, to test potential interest in a diet consisting mostly of wild greens, olive oil, whole grains, fish, vegetables, and yoghurt. Traditional local fare, by contrast, comprises high-calorie starches fried in animal fat along with bacon, cornbread, fried potatoes, and soup beans.

Her success was epistemological rather than practical.

It was commonly assumed that her menu offering would be rejected flat out on cultural grounds, with people declaring they could never convince their relatives to eat such foods and anyway didn't know how to cook them. But no. Locals liked the proposed menu, but noted they had limited access to its ingredients and that they cost too much. The other worry was about how some of the foods perish quickly, given the distance traveled for shopping and the fact that one in three local jobs were actually in another country, creating household-management-time pressures.

In short, a foray into the field reminded the public health official that, in her words, "unless people believe they have the ability to achieve the desired results, they may have little or no incentive to act."

Circle the policy wagons

Information from the field that upsets hypotheses is normally precious in science, but is often just exasperating to policy-makers. And so in very many ways, the current turn in the nutrition arena is to react to failed outreach initiatives by discarding educational campaigns to change habits in general and instead going for a wholesale overhaul of the source of the citizens' food chain. Hence the current calls for sugar consumption levels to be cut drastically, a move that imposes hefty costs on food manufacturers, be it through lost sales or by product reformulations, that will eventually pop up at the cash register.

This is a process driven by what University of Limerick professor Lee Monaghan astutely terms "obesity epidemic entrepreneurs," a varied cast of characters who together work to position obesity as a correctable problem to which they have the answers. For the campaigners, commercial weight-loss centers and curative products to succeed, spadework has to be done by members of the scientific community and amplified by the media, according to Monaghan, who has done ethnographic fieldwork at for-profit slimming clubs across the UK. A synoptic version of his model would start with the enshrinement of the BMI index, proceed to high-level declarations of "war against obesity," and induce journalists to embrace a seemingly noble cause. Then politicians will nudge regulators into producing a "deliverable."[11] The sugar warriors appear to be making reasonable headway, although victories so far may be Pyrrhic.

In July 2015, the UK's Scientific Advisory Committee on Nutrition (SACN), delivered its highly-awaited *Carbohydrates and Health* report to the government, 24 years since the previous set of guidelines. It recommended that free sugars – including that contained in honey – account for no more than five percent of daily energy intake.

The US government is currently asking for input on new dietary guidelines scheduled for release in late 2015. The advisory committee kept its recommendation for sugar to be capped at 10 percent of dietary intake, while noting the promise of microbiome science and suggesting that more frequent family meals might help weight control by cutting down on adolescent screen time. It also observed that Americans don't eat enough vegetables.[12]

SACN's decision, presuming it is accepted by the government, seems like, and largely is, a wholesale victory for Action on Sugar and the phalanx of researchers who have decried sugar as a short cut to an early death.

So is the fat lady going too sing now?

The curious thing about the 300-page SACN report, though, is that it fully exonerated sugar from its alleged crimes regarding the slew of unwelcome medical conditions its enemies have claimed. It concluded there was no association between sugar and coronary events, diastolic blood pressure, fasting total HDL or LDL cholesterol concentrations, fasting triacylglycerol concentration, fasting blood glucose, blood insulin, nor Type 2 diabetes mellitus. For good measure, pure fructose was also sees as unrelated to diabetes.

So what was sugar's crime? There is evidence that sugar boosts dietary energy intake.

Drum roll, please! Sugar is caloric, and excess calories lead to weight gain. The precise story, in SACN's words, is that people in an ad libitum state do not compensate for energy delivered as sugar by reducing their intake of other foods.[13] In short, sugar is naughty because we are naughty, not because of any specific metabolic or dietary quality it has. Now you know.

Just to be clear, the SACN itself cited a mathematical formula to explain that its decision was based on a plan to cut daily energy intake by 100 calories a day per person and acknowledged that downsizing sugar intake was "one approach" to achieve that. But instead of urging people to cut 100 calories – about ten potato chips – the government was instructed to focus on sugar. Cups of tea will become rare treats or amount to furtive cheating.

While obesity epidemic entrepreneurs rejoiced, there has been no public reaction to the SACN report's declaration that it did see an association between diabetes and both white rice and potatoes. No recommendations were forthcoming on those two staple foods because in the committee's opinion the amount of rice triggering the problem is atypical of most contemporary British diets, and because with potatoes it may depend on the way they are cooked. SACN also ordered up a sharp increase in the daily intake of dietary fibers – the kind that our gut microbes like – raising its "daily reference value" to 30 grams a day, a 25 percent increase from the previous recommendation and in fact higher than what had previously been posited as the maximum desired amount. Acquiring those fibers really ought not to be done by eating more carbohydrates in the form of breads, cereal, or pasta, as that would negate the 100-calorie reduction that is apparently the point of the exercise. That leaves fruit and vegetables. The new guidelines amount to a big regulatory push that will require up to doubling the daily outlay for the most expensive food types.

The obesity epidemic entrepreneurs didn't mention that.

Some commercial food products may be reformulated to reduce their sugar count, although it can be a delicate process as sugar carries out various technical functions such as offsetting acidity in tomato sauce and allowing ice cream to solidify at lower temperatures. An easier option for breakfast cereals is to substitute starch in order to maintain texture, which would incidentally restore the caloric load.

You might think that individuals might each find their own appropriate way to slash 100 calories, perhaps by cutting toast, or by getting some exercise. Nope. The obesity epidemic entrepreneurs have that escape route clearly covered, as demonstrated by a kerfuffle that made page one of *The New York Times* in August 2015 and was widely reprinted around the world.

Pointless exercise

The case warrants a closer look, as it provides an example of the amplification stage of the entrepreneurial process. Three American professors announced in a prominent professional journal in March that Coca-Cola was funding them and some international colleagues to set up the Global Energy Balance Network (GEBN), which aimed to focus attention on "both sides" of the energy balance equation, code for the potential role of physical exercise in the matter of overweight and obesity. They noted that a Google search indicated a 70-fold difference in the number of articles about diet and obesity compared to those discussing physical activity's role.

The professors are all known for their work in this field, but Coca-Cola Inc.'s sole initial sponsorship of the "network" – and its clumsy hosting of the apposite website – was depicted as a devilish piece of propaganda aimed at "shifting blame" for obesity away from bad diets.[14] Corporate spin in science is naturally a worry, but corporate funding appears very well entrenched. Indeed, David Ludwig, a Harvard professor who has loudly linked sodas and childhood obesity for years, heads an obesity prevention center fruitfully funded by a foundation set up by New Balance, the sportswear brand, while the Bill and Melinda Gates Foundation, one of the biggest sponsors of nutrition initiatives in the world, has held large stake in so-called Big Food companies as well as in the retail giants that distribute their wares.

GEBN, for its part, did not just recruit craven jocks. Its European representative is Arne Astrup, head of the University of Copenhagen's 150-strong nutrition department and an active sponsor of the New Nordic Diet. Somewhat of a polymath and a heavy hitter in the nutrition field, Astrup – who advises a number of companies including Novo Nordisk, the world's largest producer of insulin – has authored research arguing that inadequate sleep may trigger diabetes. Astrup's name wasn't mentioned in the storm of controversy.

Anyway, to underscore the scandal, *Times* reporter Anahad O'Connor cited a paper reviewing 17 studies specifically on sodas which found those funded by big brands tended to play up the lack of proof of any adverse health outcomes while the others actively hypothesized a link between sodas and weight gain. The issue in the end boiled down to the idea that Coca-Cola, a longtime sponsor of exercise initiatives, aimed to thwart regulatory momentum against its products by buying ideological space.

Standard fare – but *The Times*' language was rich in political nuance, suggesting that "independent public health experts" are consensually in agreement that physical activity cannot offset calories and proceeding to refer to sugary drinks as "high glycemic foods." Coca-Cola's glycemic index, a measure the SACN found to be of negligible clinical importance, is not particularly high. A can clocks in well below the level of a bagel or a baguette, or 50 percent less than a four-ounce serving of frozen Tofu.[15]

While *The New York Times* story was primarily about an alleged conflict of interest, it inevitably allied with Action on Sugar's obesity epidemic entrepreneurs. As it happens, the organization's science director, Dr. Malhotra, had already responded to Blair's announcement of the GEBN project by writing in the same *British Journal of Sports Medicine* that physical activity's relation to obesity was a "myth" and working in both an allegation that Coca-Cola was using the tactics of the tobacco industry and a pitch for higher consumption of fat. The editorial, along with Dr. Malhotra's statement to the BBC that obese people must only eat less and not do an iota of exercise, triggered a wave of criticism for sending what one top UK public health official termed an "idiotic" message. Amusingly, the online editorial had to be briefly suspended due to an undeclared conflict of interest by one of the co-authors.[16]

Why *The Times* got involved in the cat fight is a bit of a mystery, not least as the study the newspaper cited actually reported that the college-educated white men with an average BMI over 29 who were its main subjects had managed to shed a reasonable 3.9 kilograms or more than eight pounds in a year after an hour a day on the treadmill. Moreover, they added lean tissue while shedding fat cells, which is widely understood to set the stage for further weight loss down the line.[17] Even weirder, the science behind the idea that physical exercise won't lead to weight loss also implies that people who drink less soda after a targeted tax on beverages will lose much less weight than its champions promise![18]

At any rate, soon going to the gym will not be necessary, as scientists have just synthesized a molecule they say can trick cells into thinking the body has been exercising, triggering weight-slashing metabolic responses in obese people. That sounds easier![19]

The *Times'* purported scoop was published at the same time as *The Economist* published an article noting a huge uptick in the number of Americans working out, weightlifting or engaged in training exercise today compared to 2003 – the same year that US obesity peaked. Physical exercise has become a pastime for 60 percent of the richest fifth of Americans, who often spend up to $50 an hour at gym clubs, compared to 40 percent a dozen years ago, while rates increased modestly for the middle classes as well. Only the poorest fifth opted to cut back on yoga and aerobics classes.

That the obesity epidemic entrepreneurs engage in abstract squabbles over exactly which preventive theory is the best universal answer to a complex problem, while actual people respond to their own needs, often status-driven and with some lacking access to the required facilities, may be a persistent trait for public health discourse in general. According to Lars Thorup Larsen, the whole idea that prevention is better than treatment has not in fact led to any savings and risks becoming a perverse interpretation of the famous claim that it was nutrition and not medical treatment that led to the major drops in mortality reported in nineteenth-century Britain.

That thesis, made by Thomas McKeown, argued that improved social conditions rather than science and policy led to better lives. Bureaucrats now embrace it as showing that lifestyle changes are the key health drivers. Larsen says that amounts to a "colossal leap of faith" as the thesis itself argues that the historical changes of the 1800s were nothing to do with individualist lifestyle choices but rather better housing and broader access to more food.

Very often "policy learning" is not connected to objective experience but amounts to an interpretation of previous policy experience – just as lobbyists on both sides of the sugar debate may be tempted to learn from the tobacco wars, which themselves were mostly carried out after smoking's peak, just as London's anti-gin laws came as locals were tiring of the stuff anyway.

"It is the epistemology of prevention – and not the intention nor the actors involved – that is problematic, because it often leaps all too quickly from tangible or measurable health problems to believing it can fix them," Larsen observes. The peculiar culture of public health entrepreneurs, he concludes, is their penchant to use statistical descriptions of preventable factors in society as pointing to lifestyle while ignoring factors like economy, education, taste, or culture, on which actual lifestyles depend.[20]

Sounding mathematical alarm

One way to rein in the gap between policy and practice might be to require that, in cases of failure to achieve progress on a given goal, policy-makers be explicitly required either to double down on the material efforts to achieve that goal, or to acknowledge it is not a priority. Thus if a political leader promises to put a chicken in every pot but the fowl do not arrive, she or he is not allowed to pledge three chickens in every pot. That might boost accountability and lead to more sober claims on all sides about the economic costs and savings of various problems and their proposed solutions.

Consider *Healthy People 2010*, the US government's guideline health agenda, which was promulgated in 2000 with goals for the decade ahead. One of its 20 itemized pledges related to nutrition was to assure that half of all Americans "consume at least three daily servings of vegetables, with at least one-third being dark green or orange vegetables." The final review of the overall 2010 document, issued in 2013, headlined by claiming mission accomplished or at least progress made on 71 percent of the 733 goals monitored. The midterm report on the new *Healthy People 2020* suggests things are going even better as it cites fewer than 12 percent of its key indicators moving away from its goals.[21]

But a cursory look shows that the vegetable benchmark flatlined at a tiny percent. Still, that was counted as a success story among the twenty nutritional objectives, 16 of which moved in the wrong direction, including child, adolescent, and adult obesity rates, which instead of falling rose by more than 50 percent.

Prevalence of diabetes also rose by half instead of falling by a third. This target was shelved in *Healthy People 2020*, which opted instead to aim to lower "total mortality" among those with the disease.

That's a noble aim, and will be easier to achieve as it has been declining since at least 2000. But it reflects treatment, not preventive policies. (Interestingly, the target of increasing those engaged in physical exercise has already reached its 2020 target.)

In the wake of public confusion over the recent reversal of forty years of official recommendations to avoid eating fats, it may be important for nutrition experts to stave off a credibility crisis. Arguing over whether added sugars should be reduced to 5 percent – or how about 3 percent! – of total dietary energy intake may seem to consumers as boring inside baseball if progress on the previous longstanding recommendation still has a long way to go.

"Inflated promises unlikely to be filled" and not effectively monitored is a recipe for the government to promote "myth-based policies," says Michael Marlow, a professor of economics at California Polytechnic University, warning that the disinclination to examine alternative explanations "explain[s] why so little progress has been made on the obesity front." Despite rhetorical emphasis on nutrition being seen in holistic terms, practical focus on line-item targets can lead to paradoxical situations where achieving one may entail trashing another. A brewing problem on that front is that the government's own research suggests that the call to eat less sugar and more vegetables may add calories and will – especially those dark green or orange ones – add sodium to diets, thus contradicting another cardiovascular goal.

The mechanical solution is to use less salt in processing and cooking food, but just as the war on chocolate milk led to school-age children abandoning calcium in favor of soda, insisting on a shift to vegetables while at the same time denying the main ingredient that makes them more palatable to many people could easily backfire.

Intellectually, that can be written off as reflecting cultural notions of palatability, or well-known bad habits. But apparently it's part of a global problem wherein the recommendations hammered out in the smoke-free but perhaps windowless rooms of the food commissars simply do not add up. Drewnowski looked at flagship data from the US, the UK, France and Mexico and found "close to zero" compliance in meeting at the same time both the WHO guidelines for sodium and potassium intake, and that doing so does not appear feasible.[22]

One approach, endorsed by Action on Sugar's elder sibling, Action on Salt, has been adopted by the UK, which has set a target to cut salt consumption by 60 percent through 2025, which is quite a challenge for chefs, home cooks, and food manufacturers alike. But Action on Potassium has yet to be set up. As it happens, the foods that pack that vital ingredient tend to be more expensive, and some of them, notably fish, face sustainability restraints as it is. But more to the point, it's not clear how people will eat these potassium-rich foods without adding salt.[23]

"There is a case to be made for more feasibility research in the formulation of public policy," says Drewnowski, anticipating major levels of non-compliance ahead and adding that those prescribing diets need to suggest ways they can be afforded.

As for WHO's 5 percent line on added sugars, the model diets proposed by the US government as healthy are at least mathematically compatible. However, it is tight – people will have to cut out orange juice and can have only two aspartame-based desserts a week, and forget about cranberries, according to Joanne Slavin, a nutritionist who sat on the dietary guidelines committee in 2010. "It would seem doubtful for the American population to sustain a diet that does not allow for even small treats in their daily routine," she said.

8 A Wild Bias

Instead of dirt and poison we have rather chosen to fill our hives with honey and wax; thus furnishing mankind with the two noblest of things, which are sweetness and light.

Jonathan Swift

I personally don't take sugar with my coffee, and consider an appreciation of bitter tastes a trait to be encouraged. It's a great complement to our primordial evolutionary instinct to equate sweetness with edibility.

I assumed sugar, which I never eat on its own, was a moderate vice. One morning I was gently chiding my daughter for her inordinate, in my view, consumption of a popular breakfast cookie that was clearly made of hyper-refined grains and gobs of sugar. The hope was to coax her to diversify into muesli, the no-logo discount toasted European granola I was then eating with unsweetened yogurt.

We checked the nutrition labels. My breakfast had fewer calories, slightly more fiber and, to my amazement, significantly more sugar. There are "natural" alternatives, but the one I most like represents a lifestyle issue as it costs more than three times as much. I had seen headlines about soda taxes and toxic sugar, but "advanced glycation end products" packs a punch without even using an adjective.

I needed to learn, so I immersed myself in science and nutrition themes. I'm used to the idea that things aren't what they seem and am of the view that you can learn a lot from a French and an Italian judge at a wine and cheese contest, but it might not be about wine or cheese.

The same goes for opinion polls, so given there's a policy debate about sugar I looked at a few of those.

It turns out, as many local referenda have now shown, that people don't like sugar taxes, which seem to jar with notions of individual choice, while labeling requirements are generally supported. Some polls are of quite high quality in their design. I wouldn't have guessed, for example, that people who think obesity is caused by genetic factors tend not to support a policy intervention, on the grounds that it seems pointless. And I was curious to learn the nuances of why people might think there is an obesogenic environment out there and how that should be addressed.

What struck me, then, is that most of the polls embed a negative portrayal of sugar, and especially soft drinks, in their questions. The survey aims to test the political air, whereas I actually just wanted to know whether the premise was accurate. One of the best academic exercises, led by a Yale University epidemiologist, mentioned that portrayal of obesity as an epidemic is galvanized by people's fears about downward mobility in general, which seems cogent. The paper concluded, though, by offering advice: advocates of public obesity prevention policies should frame their project with low-blame metaphors and play up the idea of industry manipulation, while those interested in blocking the use of public policy should play up concepts of sloth, gluttony, and individual responsibility. Other polls of this sort, usually funded by tax-exempt universities and foundations, have shown that referring to diabetes rather than obesity greatly boosts public interest in governmental action.[1]

Those are astute observations about strategic communications, and give some traction as to how the news media might have a role. By and large, apparently, pro-soda-tax arguments are twice as frequent as anti-tax arguments, academics are the main source of the former, and alleged health benefits are four times as likely to be mentioned as the likelihood that such a tax would be levied most heavily on the poor.[2]

There's little mention of whether the scientific premise that sugar is somehow to blame for obesity or diabetes holds water, nor of the prospective function of other sweeteners, which is surprising given there's evidently also some unease about aspartame and quite a lot of research going on into finding super-sweet alternatives sources for our food system. In terms of framing the debate, "Big Food" appears to have lost the battle against quicker-witted and bigger public health entrepreneurs.

But it all seemed kind of self-referential. Sometimes the frame doesn't matter at all. I was very amused to hear that Telluride, a ski town of 2,000 probably pretty healthy and wealthy people in my home state of Colorado, even voted on a soda tax, and yet they slugged it out. My favorite bit was a realpolitik advocate who suggested the vacation resort might gain some free international publicity if it became the first to pass such a levy. More relevant, perhaps, was that many voters disliked the out-of-state funding that allowed a paid campaign manager in favor of the initiative. Big Lobby isn't always a business story, apparently. Anyway, it didn't pass.

And they often don't, nor do rules for labels on genetically-modified foods, even though one might have expected the opposite from all the chatter.

Peering deeper it turned out that the science is not so clear, which is odd given the thousands of papers that have been published on the sugar question, mostly accusatory.

Frustration at not clinching the case may explain the proliferation of so many new theories about diabesity. Given that the problem is increasingly billed as a global one, I made a point of seeking out information from beyond the beltway.

One of my favorites comes from India, and maps the molecular machinery through which insulin resistance emerges as the result of aggression control, increasingly required in an urbanized world. A few days in the woods engaged in "neuro-motor actions characteristic of Stone Age hunting or combat" led to notable declines in key inflammatory markers among 19 Indian diabetics.[3]

I stumbled onto one highly articulate and funny argument that the old sloth-and-gluttony tropes are in fact solid, as metabolic syndrome is a lethal punishment designed to uphold food security among primitive bands. It's evolution's way of giving the boot to people when they start bringing in less food or eat more than their share.[4] That's a variant on the "thrifty gene" hypothesis, which argues that we were kitted out to hunt and gather in a harsh and fluctuating world, and adapting to round-the-clock supply of processed foods is biologically trying.

Some Canadian researchers suggest that obesity may not be a pathology at all but an a priori biological adaptation to the abundance of endocrine-disrupting insecticides and pesticides. The body develops fatty tissue precisely to absorb and insulate these from the rest of the body, a self-protecting gambit that defers death. Tests have shown high traces of specific chemicals known as persistent organic pollutants, many now illegal but widely used after 1950, in obese patients' blood plasma, in young diabetic Mexicans, and in Greek and Indian mothers of low-birth weight children.[5]

The microbiome studies are perhaps the most paradigm-busting of them all, much like the germ theory once was, or the important realization that diseases such as beriberi were in fact due to deficiencies rather than surfeits or pathogens. The mainstream show, though, consists of scientists who run rats through their paces and isolate processes that appear to be adverse. I admit my intellectual allegiance, or limit, makes me wary of a model-based episteme that by design cannot cope with the interactivity that observation itself instigates.

Then there's the data, and what to make of it. Is there an obesity problem? Yes, but it may not be as huge as portrayed. Is there a diabetes problem? The disease is rightly often called a syndrome and the implicit "rift" is widespread, but naturally multifactorial. The correlation studies are important, but there are a lot of them, and those pegged to lack of sleep or C-sections tell as good an obesity story as does the rise of HFCS. So little is known about the thousands of industrial chemicals and pollutants and food additives – which vastly outnumber the kinds of basic foods we eat! – that there will no doubt be more fascinating correlation studies to come one day, and perhaps even a clincher.

All of this leaves much ambiguity around the nutrition message. I have been told repeatedly about the problem that it is all but impossible to do a randomized controlled trial with a sufficiently large number of people over many years. It's not just the ethical quandary, but also the time factor. More than a millennium passed since the fall of Rome before the mere formulation of the hypothesis that a prime cause was lead poisoning.

Correlations have at any rate led, through the newish idea of epigenetics – wherein environmental factors somehow transmit back into genetic functions – to the idea of the metabolic ghetto, which offers compelling insight into the historic pathways of malnutrition. And now evidence that a single fecal transplant can induce obesity suggests that the role of diet may be completely different from conventional models, themselves of fairly recent vintage given that the idea of a vitamin is less than a century old.

The public, meanwhile, is told to avoid fats, then carbohydrates, then sugar, and now told not to bother to exercise. Purgatory is a useful concept for getting by in the meantime. Or perhaps, like the folks Orwell visited in Wigan Pier who insisted on white bread, people keep to their relatively new traditions because standardized and branded foods are a remembrance of the widespread debauchment to which they were proposed as a response. I've read at least one bit of marketing research saying people will not eat vegetables until these too are branded.

The recommendation to eat what one's great-grandmother ate has, after all, a rather terrifying aspect. Milk in Matthew Arnold's London contained about 25 percent added water. In Italy, adulteration of olive oil was widespread at the time, as discovered and denounced by one of the newly-unified country's first parliamentary inquiries. In nearby France wine was regularly spiked with added sugars to achieve high alcohol content in order to lower tax levies when it was shipped to Paris and other cities, after which it was watered down again for retail sale.[6] Such a rampant case of added sugars is a core practice today in making champagne. Politely known as "chaptalization," it is still done when grapes have low sugar content, at least in France. It is illegal in Italy and California. The eminently modifiable practice done in the name of profitability does not appear to reflect lifestyle choices, though, but rather temperature patterns.

Fortunately, weddings can still be celebrated with prosecco as, with all due respect to stainless steel tanks, the Italian bubbly contains only naturally occurring rather than added sugars. But surely it is a pity to see champagne – which Brillat-Savin noted can make you do silly things – shunted into history's rubbish bin because a caged and bored quasi-mutant rat got sick on a diet of fructose and crumbled Oreos. No doubt an exception will be made, as it was in Hogarth's time, when gin was demonized but expensive wine was not. Demanding that champagne be reformulated doesn't sound like a wise communications strategy. And that's the rub: why aren't all sugars equal?

It seems that sugar is a matter of taste: my kind is okay, yours not so much. We should probably embrace that rather than be annoyed.

Simplicity and rapidification

We are facing a deficiency, not a surplus, and my view is that wild plants can help us, both biologically through the microbiome, and through less tangible channels – because if we can find the time and space to forage, that's already a sign of lower stress. Not so long ago, most people knew how to find and use them, and this may be one of the biggest differences from today.

Consider purslane.

Portulaca oleracea is many things. Called "little hogweed," it is on the US Department of Agriculture's hit list as an invasive, noxious weed, and gardeners across the country curse its ground-covering tenacity, deep roots, and the vast number of seeds it casts to take over more soil. A fleshy succulent weed that deploys C4 photosynthesis, it was brought to North America on purpose and is named in a cookbook given as a wedding gift to George Washington's wife, Martha. It was also cited by Pliny the Elder for its health-giving properties and has long been used in Chinese and Mexican traditional medicine as a treatment for diabetes. When it was given to laboratory rats a few years ago it led to weight loss, lower blood glucose levels, and improved insulin flows.[7]

Its virtues are strong omega-3 fatty acids, the kind that are usually expensive, plenty of vitamin C and D, high potassium content and abundant glutathione, an effective antioxidant that acts potently with our gut microbes. It is spinach plus avocado plus asparagus with a dash of olive and fish oil – a superfood, if you can stomach the texture and sour taste. It is very much like watercress, once a staple of the English countryside and still ordered in by working-class Londoners until the late 1800s.

Purslane is prolific, and probably growing on the edges of a neighbor's driveway right now. So why aren't we eating it? Well, while some people sing its praises, most agree with Job in the Bible, who described it as "slimy." It's pretty much the opposite of an Advanced Glycation Endproduct and has to be boiled for ages or eaten raw, in which case sparingly or with yoghurt to dampen down some of its less salubrious contents. Mostly it's been forgotten. Hopping out and grabbing some wild strands as a condiment for meals was common in Greece and southern Italy in the 1960s, when Ancel Keys coined the profitable concept of the Mediterranean diet and hailed the variant on Crete as the healthiest in the world. Today, 86 percent of the people in rural Crete are overweight, far more than the USA, and there is no evidence the sugar supply went into orbit – in fact calorie intakes have declined. Fast food has taken a modest hold on the island, but those looking for a culprit in the dietary data will end up scrutinizing the threefold rise in meat, a surge in potatoes, and a 10-fold jump in vegetable oils other than olive oil.

But if we look for what has gone missing, another picture emerges.

Consumption of wine, a known provider of phenols for the microbiome, has fallen by half. And all the meat and cheaper oils suggest that hefty consumption of raw plants such as purslane, once a signature trait and nearly daily table fixture on the island, has declined. As a foraged item it is naturally absent from official statistics.[8]

The role of wild greens in Crete is often mentioned in adulatory terms today, popping up on tourist sites, but with all due respect for identity politics the startling increase in obesity strongly suggests this is nostalgia. Indeed, recent claims that island residents still seek edible plants are full of quotes from elderly ladies who say the habit was born during wartime famine and young people don't do it anymore.[9] The same is true for Italy, where researchers trying to identify traditionally eaten wild plants find themselves interviewing aficionados aged 70 or over. Ethnobotanists find the same across Europe, although knowledge is fresher in places such as Albania which were isolated until twenty years ago.

That said, keystone phytochemical suppliers were a vital part of pre-industrial diets around the world. Acorns, once well known to the Pima, are an example. They can take a lot of time to beat into edibility. Our cave-dwelling ancestors in Morocco 15,000 years ago had time, and the archeological evidence suggests they used a lot of it to prepare acorns – eating so many they developed rampant dental caries.

With modern grains, cultivation techniques and yields have been massively improved, but we mill out 80 percent of the nutrients in order that the flour is dry and has a shelf life. The same is true of sugar. Indeed, sugar cane juice is commonly billed as a supernutrient today for its high calcium, potassium, zinc, and magnesium content and antioxidants on par with pure phenolic acids. Interesting research is being done now on how to recuperate these elements.[10]

Whether there is a way for them to be integrated with refined sugar is a question for engineers, who may find solutions to a practical task faster than public policy can find them for complex multi-factorial social problems. The key point will be that many food recipes and techniques require sugar to be pure. Consider the meringue, first known as "white biskit bread" in an English cookbook from 1604. These are treats that last, but a soggy meringue is called a weeping one.

The main reason for refining grains and sugar is to achieve dryness. That means the fiber factor is lost, but these staple foods are very rarely eaten alone so the assumption is fiber will be picked up elsewhere. Sugar's case is particularly extreme, as residual moisture content above 0.04 percent is ruinous. Yet Marcel Proust would never have been able to dunk his *petite madeleine* in tea and overcome the "vicissitudes of life" in 3,000 pages of memories without sugar.

Indeed, it was when a way to make dry sugar granules was discovered in India that humans first harnessed *Saccharum officinarum*'s special photosynthetic powers in a way allowing the conquest of space, through transportability, and time, through preservation.

In a strong sense, then, sugar was a co-conspirator in setting the stage for metabolic rift, or what Pope Francis, in his 2015 encyclical on the environment "*Laudato Si*," called "rapidification." That's a word he coined and refers to a process whereby Cretans forget to pick purslane and Americans invent plastic cup holders to make it easier to consume high-energy foods and drinks with one hand while driving a car.[11] Rapidification is when human activity outraces the pace of biology. It can work wonders but also, the pontiff observed, become a "source of anxiety."

The chronic stress today's lifestyle engenders has become our main predator. One of its more insidious stalking habits, prolonged cortisol disorder, also stokes irregular sleeping patterns. Some 40 percent of Americans say they usually sleep for six hours or less, a fourfold increase from 1942 and a shift that was largely complete by 1990. Official data also show sharp drops in average sleep among Chinese and American children, suggesting that rapidification processes can start early.

And lo, chronic sleep disturbance of the kind associated with night-shift work for five years or more demonstrably led to higher BMI and jumps of 50 percent to 100 percent in diabetic outcomes in large-scale studies done in Finland, Belgium as well as in Italy and Japan, both countries whose local dietary habits are often lauded for their cardiovascular benefits.[12] One calculation found that the risk of obesity declined by 30 percent for every extra hour of sleep, which inverted means it rises by about half for every hour less. Another recent study found a net 677 calorie difference – equal to five cans of Coca-Cola – in daily calorie intake due to sleep restriction.[13]

And that's not all. New research suggests that a single night of sleep loss works havoc on our internal cellular clocks and already starts to produce lasting genetic changes of a kind that impairs glucose tolerance, the medical marker of the path to obesity and diabetes. Adverse gene methylation patterns were visible in the adipose tissue of young and athletic Swedish men the morning after sleep deprivation. It was known that one bad night reduces insulin sensitivity, but that can be reversed with rest, whereas less is known about bodily programming.[14] To its credit, the US Centers for Disease Protection Control and Prevention did try in 2014 to brand insufficient sleep as a public health epidemic, noting that it causes obesity and diabetes as well as increases traffic crashes, hospital errors, and industrial disasters, but the proclamation has so far been ignored.[15] One reason may be that it is hard to be a sleep deficit entrepreneur. Products already exist for that, such as coffee, energy drinks, and soda, as well as a substantial array of licit and illicit drugs.

Still, it is curious that the public health activists aren't all over this obesogenic factor. It has a corporate angle, especially in retail, a rapidly globalizing sector which runs the places where people buy most of their food and increasingly has Big Food by the throat. Moreover, a solution would likely bolster dietary guidelines by bolstering collective meals instead of advanced rapidification end products such as snacks.[16]

Add together estimates for weight gain due to the decline in smoking, sleep deficits, and C-sections, toss in a bit for sedentarism despite the howls, add at least a bit more for air pollution, environmental chemicals, antidepressant and antibiotics usage, give a hat tip to the metabolic ghetto effect, and there's not a lot of room left in the metabolic jailhouse for ordinary sugar.

An epistemic coda

The reason, I venture, that sugar and in particular sweetened beverages are the target of dietary reformers is because, given the wickedness of obesity and metabolic syndrome, they are seen as simpler and faster. Call it the "candy is dandy but liquor is quicker" thesis: an upstream regulatory intervention aimed at curbing the entry of sugar into the industrial food chain amounts to an end run of all the time-consuming interactions required to implement viable educational programs, usher in changed maternity ward, farming and labor practices, and all the complications of monitoring so-called voluntary plans engaging Big Food itself as a player in the forging of a solution.[17]

Such a single-shot approach seems dangerous. We could after all also decide to deal with the complexity of our gut bacteria by using a big-bang dose of antibiotics followed by a standard-issue fecal implant for all to make sure everyone shares a universal microbiome, which surely would make it easier to monitor, cure, and control everyone's future health trajectories with a single template. We can even police that by using new methods to test human hair samples for C4 isotypes to see if anyone is secretly eating too much sugar, bypassing the need to talk to or even watch them.

That's not the simplicity that gets hailed as a virtue, and it makes rapidification go faster.

In noting Dr. Lustig's stalwart opposition to pleasure as any justification for sugar, I mentioned Locke's distinction between imaginary and true happiness and the implicit judgment that the latter is the special preserve of elite knowledge.

But the sweetness-and-light approach reveals that the frontiers of knowledge today all point to the importance of downstream effects crawling back up the presumed causal pathway. Everything that happens, from working the night shift to a drought in southern Arizona, ends up methylating genes linked to metabolism in a way that can over generations transform the genome itself. Thus part of our lives is not ours, and who will decide that?

"The new metabolism is no longer the interface between Man and Nature, as it was for the 19th and 20th centuries, but a metabolism for the human condition in technical society, where the food is manufactured and designed at the molecular level, the air and the water are full of the byproducts of human endeavor and manufactured environments beget different physiologies," says Hannah Landecker, a brilliant scholar working on how the rise of microbiomics and epigenetics may be understood and might be used.

In the emergent Anthropocene coming into view, there is no lord of the jungle in the microbiome, nor can there be elite knowledge in Locke's sense. Consumer marketing and public health policy are biological actors, along with parental effort and the natural resistance of youth to resist authority, all with the potential to embed social, economic, and cultural difference as much as progress.[18] Top-down rules and regulations effectively make learning unnecessary, and so despite their best intentions anti-sugar crusaders are embracing a recipe that will restrict not pleasure but access to true happiness.

Put another way, ad libitum is a risk factor, but not a disease. It is known that rats live longer if not allowed an ad libitum diet, but the issue only arises because they are not free-living but caged, and that cultural discontinuity is ultimately the unique cause of their metabolic woes.

Invocations of a "war on obesity" no doubt aspire to inculcate a state of emergency to justify a special exception to this liberal epistemology, but there is no enemy in post-industrial metabolism, which is more like jazz than computer code.

There is no past Edenic model of nutrition to revert to, and the risk of metabolic syndrome reflects the violence of rapid change on all levels, not just our diet. As for obesity, it appears already to be on a slow decline, even if it may take decades for that to become clear.

There was no policy solution to London's gin epidemic because the newly urbanized poor tired of it on their own. They shifted to well-sugared tea, unable to know that public policy was about to subject wheat, the keystone calorie source of the time, to a tax-and-supply crackdown, a decision followed shortly afterwards with a poorhouse policy dubbed the "starvation act."[19]

The focus on identifying specific causes of lethal diseases led eventually to the germ theory and the great breakthroughs of antibiotics, but at the cost of suppressing attention to the social conditions underlying the epidemics of the time.

The political, social and economic changes afoot during the Industrial Revolution led to preferring a technical etiology of disease over the social approach to medicine advocated by reformers such as Rudolf Virchow in Germany, a doctor sent to inspect a typhus epidemic in Upper Silesia in 1848. Although his expertise was in cellular pathology, he realized the outbreak had taken such heavy tolls because of the misery faced by the Polish-speaking local people, who were facing famine and poverty on top of the gradual degradation of cultural norms and hygiene due to centuries of feudal subjugation and failed application of the rules set down by far-away Prussian authorities – and so proposed "free and unlimited democracy" as the best cure.[20]

The multifaceted nature of today's epidemics and the unsettling evidence of the roles of culture and status in their genesis suggest that the best solution will lie less in a top-down one-size-fits-all rule setting sugar intake targets far below plausibly achievable levels, but in efforts to heal the metabolic rift on a broader global tableau and enable people to restore their own balance.

As things stand, sugar consumption is declining in countries that use it most, and rising where it is less common. Its efficient production of calories should be exploited for a growing world population, offering time and energy to fund a quest to boost diversity elsewhere in the food system of the Anthropocene and engineer novelties such as C4 rice to deal with climate change.

"The lack of fiber is desirable; the softer the cane, the more it is esteemed by the natives for eating," Elmer Brandes wrote after visiting Papua New Guinea to learn of new species and ancient practices. That rather sums sugar up: it is a sweet energy source, but it does not cater to our nutritional needs nor those of our gut microbes. For those who want to lose calories it is a fine place, although hardly the only place, to start. Our deeper dietary conundrum, meanwhile, is one of lack, not abundance.

This book started by talking about how high people will climb for honey and will end with a small recognition of those who make it. Sugar in the world's diet is like honeybees in world agriculture. Studies of pollination suggest that the richness or number of bee species actually matters more for farming yields than the abundance of any one dominant type. So while the honeybee is of great importance given the surprisingly sharp uptick since 1990 in the world's reliance on pollinated crops, improving conditions for wild bees is the critical issue for the biodiversity underlying our crops in the long run.

Much as Zhao, who began his research by experimenting on himself, describes our gut as comprising motley gangs of microbes rather than following strict phylum-level orders, the demise of specialist pollinators puts at risk the mutualist relations established with plants and gradually turns all species into generalists. That, alas, is typical of times of regime change and the loss of culture based on tacit reciprocity. It's a recipe for stress.

Here's a modest proposal: sugar may even be a keystone species for ad libitum culture. It is "the universal condiment that does not spoil anything," wrote Brillat-Savarin in a book on food that has never been out of print. "Its uses vary ad infinitum because they depend on peoples and individuals."

Appendix

The World's Top 12 Crops

Sugarcane today is easily the world's No.1 crop in quantity, and the tenth-largest in value terms.

By weight (tonnes)	
Sugar cane	1.91 billion
Maize	1.02 billion
Rice	741 million
Wheat	716 million
Milk	636 million
Potatoes	376 million
Vegetables	280 million
Cassava	277 million
Soybeans	276 million
Sugar beet	247 million
Tomatoes	164 million
Barley	144 million

By value by $1000 int	
Milk	198 billion
Rice	191 billion
Pig	173 billion
Beef	171 billion
Chicken	137 billion
Wheat	85.9 billion
Soybeans	69.5 billion
Maize	77.1 billion
Sugar cane	60.8 billion
Tomatoes	59.9 billion
Eggs	56.6 billion
Potatoes	49.7 billion

Sugar cane production has quadrupled since 1961

Source: UN Food and Agriculture Organization

Postscript

This book took shape during a special moment in which the author sought to stop thinking about money and start thinking about people.

By that I mean I stopped following the monetary policy aspects of the financial and euro crises, which anyway had become political, exasperating my predilection for thinking of the economy as a system of keeping one's house in order. And I started thinking more about how comforting it is that people are such a varied and motley crew.

My gut biota no doubt changed on a long and windy path from doing fieldwork among untouchable "pariah" caste in southern India in the 1990s to listening to central bankers and hedge fund managers in the noughties. It was time to ease off the fructose and up the glucose, perhaps; shift from something stimulating but not satiating to something that fuels the brain. I hope to consume both in the future, in moderation of course, and with a more balanced sucrose-like mix.

A lot of people deserve thanks. First, I have great respect for all those engaged in the sugar war, on all sides, as amid their disputes they all share the goal of improving human welfare. And I have special debts of gratitude to Liping Zhao and Richard Oster for generously sharing their time with someone more hungry than able to cook, and to my stylistically superior mental Doppelganger Stash Luczkiw for graciously reading early drafts.

Above all though, this book was both started and finished due to my mother, wife, and daughter. Their respective roles were to endow me with skepticism and conviction, push me to get on with it, and supply me with an extra dose of native curiosity. So this book is dedicated to Katharine, Lucia, and Nora for their sweetness and light.

Notes

Chapter 1

1 Another source of weight-watching pressure came with then new practice of standard-sized off-the-rack clothing. Cf. Brumberg, Joan Jacob, "Fasting Girls: The Emerging Ideal of Slenderness in American Culture", in Linda Kerber, ed., *Women's America*, Oxford University Press, 1982. Kerry Segrave expounds in great detail on this period in her *Obesity in America, 1850-1939: A History of Social Attitudes and Treatment*, published in 2008 by McFarland & Company, Jefferson, North Carolina.

2 US District Court Order Granting Defendants' Motion to Strike, Oct. 21, 2011. Case 2:11-cv-03473-CBM-MAN Document 47. The document notes that the makers of HFCS regularly use phrases such as "sugar is sugar" while the plaintiffs "allege that HCFS is a 'man-made product' that does not 'naturally occur,' making it qualitatively different from table sugar, which they allege is extracted from cane and beets. Plaintiffs also alleged that HCFS is linked to the obesity epidemic and its effect on the human body differs from that of table sugar." While the order is very preliminary, the court also declared that "a debate about the health effects of high fructose corn syrup is an issue of public interest" and, in a sign of a potential clash between federal agencies down the road, added that the court "is not persuaded that the Food and Drug Administration's position, allowing HFCS to be marketed as 'natural,' conclusively determines that CRA's statement calling HFCS natural is not false or misleading." See http://sweetsurprise.com/sites/default/files/pdf/5_Anti-SLAPP_order.pdf.

3 US FDA, "Response to Petition from Corn Refiners Association to Authorize 'Corn Sugar' as an Alternate Common or Usual Name for High Fructose Corn Syrup", May 30, 2012. The FDA did not refer to scientific terminology in defending its consideration that sugars are solid and syrups are liquid, saying that it "is consistent with the common understanding of sugar and syrup as referenced in a dictionary." It also noted that dextrose, a solid, had been commonly called corn sugar for more than thirty years. See http://www.fda.gov/AboutFDA/CentersOffices/OfficeofFoods/CFSAN/CFSANFOIAElectronicReadingRoom/ucm305226.htm.

4 Jobs in the food manufacturing sector not using sugar grew by more than 10 percent during the period under review. The job losses were attributed to greater imports of

sweetened items. Cf. "Employment Changes in U.S. Food Manufacturing: The Impact of Sugar Prices", U.S. Department of Commerce, 2006, http://trade.gov/media/Publications/pdf/sugar06.pdf.

5 Martin, Bronwen, Ji, Sunggoan, Maudsley, Stuart and Mattson Mark P., "'Control' Laboratory Rodents are Metabolically Morbid: Why it matters", *Proceedings of the National Academy of Sciences*, Vol. 107:14, pp. 6127-6133, http://www.pnas.org/content/107/14/6127.full DOI:10.1073/pnas.0912955107. The authors sharply note that wild mice live longer than laboratory mice and that laboratory rats live up to 50 percent longer if they are subjected to rations rather than ad lib access to chow pellets. They wryly note at the end that while fat rats may in fact increasingly be appropriate benchmarks for people, the normal state of both would be leaner and that should be encouraged as the control point for experiments. Gale B. Carey and Lisa C. Merrill make related points, noting that rats fed regimented meals tend to have lower body temperature, more functional small intestines, and synchronized hepatic and digestive enzymes, whereas ad lib-fed rodents often develop conditions ranging from obesity to pancreatic or thyroid tumors that are likely to affect the nature and quality of any results of research done using them. See their "Meal-Feeding Rodents and Toxicology Research", *Chemical Research in Toxicology*, 2012, Vol. 25:8, pp. 1545-1550, http://pubs.acs.org/doi/abs/10.1021/tx300109x, DOI 10.1021/tx300109x.

6 Jim Mann, professor of human nutrition and medicine at the University of Otago and a long-time member of the WHO Nutrition Guidance Expert Advisory Group that helped draft the proposed new guidelines for intake of free sugars, noted that only 68 of the 17,000 papers survived his team's application of systematic criteria regarding their scientific utility and comparability. Cf. *Bulletin of the World Health Organization*, 2014, Vol. 92:780-781, http://www.who.int/bulletin/volumes/92/11/14-031114/en/ DOI:10.2471/BLT.14.031114.

Chapter 2

[1] Kris Gunnars, CEO of Authority Nutrition, has since 2012 sought to offer readers "the truth about nutrition." His "10 Disturbing Reasons Why Sugar Is Bad for You" has had more than 700,000 views. See http://authoritynutrition.com/10-disturbing-reasons-why-sugar-is-bad/.

[2] In 2013, the American Heart Association, the American College of Cardiology and the Obesity Society released guidelines urging doctors to consider obesity a disease: http://circ.ahajournals.org/content/early/2013/11/11/01.cir.0000437739.71477.ee. The European Court of Justice in late 2014 issued a preliminary ruling in a discrimination case noting that there was no specific law regarding obesity but opening the possibility that it was a disability: http://www.bailii.org/eu/cases/EUECJ/2014/C35413.html.

[3] Cf. Rundle, Andrew, *et al.*, "Association of Childhood Obesity with Maternal Exposure to Ambient Air Polycyclic Aromatic Hydrocarbons During Pregnancy", *American Journal of Epidemiology*, 2012, http://aje.oxfordjournals.org/content/early/2012/04/13/aje.kwr455.full, DOI: 10.1093/aje/kwr455, and Jerrett, Michael, *et al.*, "Traffic-related Air Pollution and Obesity Formation in Children: A Longitudinal, Multilevel Analysis", *Environmental Health*, 2014, Vol. 13:49, DOI: 10.1186/1476-069X-13-49, http://www.ehjournal.net/content/13/1/49, and Rundle, *et al.*, "Automobile Traffic Around the Home and Attained Body Mass Index: A Longitudinal Cohort Study of Children Aged 10-18 Years", *Preventive Medicine*, 2010, Vol. 50:1, S50-S58, http://www.ncbi.nlm.nih.gov/pmc/articles/PMC4334364/, DOI: 10.1016/j.ypmed.2009.09.026.

[4] For the cited research, see: Brochu, Pierre, *et al.*, "Physiological Daily Inhalation Rates for Health Risk Assessment in Overweight/Obese Children, Adults, and Elderly", *Risk Analysis*, 2014, Vol. 34:3, pp. 567-582, http://onlinelibrary.wiley.com/doi/10.1111/risa.12125/abstract DOI: 10.1111/risa.12125, and Irigaray, P. "Ex Vivo Study of Incorporation into Adipocytes and Lipolysis-inhibition Effect of Polycyclic Aromatic Hydrocarbons", *Toxicology Letters*, 2009, Vol. 187:1, pp. 35-39, http://www.ncbi.nlm.nih.gov/pubmed/19429241 DOI: 10.1016/j.toxlet.2009.01.021, and Whitmee, Sarah *et al.* and Clark, Lara P. *et al.*, "Safeguarding Human Health in the Anthropocene Epoch: Report of The Rockefeller Foundation/*Lancet* Commission on planetary health", *The Lancet*, 2015, http://www.thelancet.com/journals/lancet/article/PIIS0140-6736(15)60901-1/fulltext, DOI:10.1016/S0140-6736(15)60901-1, and "National Patterns in Environmental Injustice and Inequality: Outdoor NO2 Air Pollution in the United States", *PlosOne*, 2014, http://journals.plos.org/plosone/article?id=10.1371/journal.pone.0094431, DOI: 10.1371/journal.pone.0091917, and Zou, Bin *et al.*, "Spatial Cluster Detection of Air Pollution Exposure Inequities Across the United States", *PlosOne*, 2014, http://journals.plos.org/plosone/article?id=10.1371/journal.pone.0091917, DOI: 10.1371/journal.pone.0091917.

[5] A tangential note is in order here. Some people may note that the state of Colorado tends to be home to relatively low obesity levels. This author's childhood home does in fact have the lowest obesity level in the USA, but it's still 21.3 percent and up threefold since 1990. Moreover, as a mountainous state Colorado ought to have lower obesity, as the vast literature on what correlates with obesity includes a finding that residing at 3,000 meters above sea level reduces obesity risk by a factor of five compared to living below 500 meters above sea level. Cf. Voss, J.D., *et al.*, "Association of Elevation, Urbanization and Ambient Temperature with Obesity Prevalence in the United States",

International Journal of Obesity, 2013, Vol. 37, pp. 1407-1412, http://www.nature.com/ijo/journal/v37/n10/pdf/ijo20135a.pdf.

[6] "We try to be like Boy Scouts and prepared", a man in Seattle told a reporter while explaining how his family used its garage to stockpile energy bars. He said some of these bars can be heated in a toaster oven whereupon "it tastes less like a snack and more like a meal." Households earning more than $100,000 a year are the primary consumers of the more than 1,000 different "nutrition bars" on the market now. Cf. Dizik, Alina, "Snack Bars Push the Price Envelope and Find Consumers Don't Push Back", *Wall Street Journal*, June 9, 2015.l

[7] The 2014 report, *How the World Could Better Fight Obesity*, formulates a chart analyzing how much various measures would cost in disability-adjusted life years (DALYs) if implemented in the UK. Prices of these so-called DALYs ranged from $31,000 for active transport interventions to a mere $50 for "media restrictions." The report is accessible at www.mckinsey.com/insights/economic_studies/how_the_world_could_better_fight_obesity.

[8] Cf. "Effects of Diabetes Definition on Global Surveillance of Diabetes Prevalence and Diagnosis: A Pooled Analysis of 96 Population-based Studies with 331 288 Participants", *The Lancet*, 2015, http://www.thelancet.com/journals/landia/article/PIIS2213-8587(15)00129-1/fulltext DOI:10.1016/S2213-8587(15)00129-1, and Schwartz, L.M. and Woloshin, S., "Changing Disease Definitons; Implications for Disease Prevalence", *Effective Clinical Practice*, 1999, Vol. 2:2, pp..76-85, http://www.ncbi.nlm.nih.gov/pubmed/10538480.

[9] Cf. Ogden, Cynthia, *et al.*, "Prevalence of Childhood and Adult Obesity in the United States, 2011-2012", *JAMA*, 2014, Vol. 311: pp. 806-814, http://jama.jamanetwork.com/article.aspx?articleid=1832542, DOI: 10.1001/jama.2014.732. The lead author, Cynthia Ogden, is an epidemiologist at the US Center for Disease Control and Prevention who has noted that the prevalence of obesity has been basically stable for women and girls since 1999, while rising significantly for men and boys. She also notes that there is a school of thought backed by the Endocrine Society that recommends measuring children with a system that would classify as obese those in the ninety-fifth percentile of the BMI range for their age, and as overweight those with a BMI in the eighty-fifth percentile or above. Using such a metric would mean that one in twenty kids is always defined obese. See Flegal, Katharine M. and Ogden, Cynthia L., "Childhood Obesity: Are We All Speaking the Same Language?", *Advances in Nutrition*, 2011, Vol. 2:2, pp. 159s-169s, http://www.ncbi.nlm.nih.gov/pmc/articles/PMC3065752/, DOI 10.3945/an.111.000307.

[10] In this paper, Roland Sturm sees the primary cause for rising obesity as having been fueled by the fact that "Americans now have the cheapest food available in history" as a share of income. Cf. Sturm, R. *et al.*, "Obesity and Economic Environments", *A Cancer Journal for Clinicians*, 2014, Vol 64:5, pp. 337-50, http://www.ncbi.nlm.nih.gov/pubmed/24853237, DOI: 10.3322/caac.21237. His colleague Deborah Cohen says the "hidden influences" behind the obesity crisis rely on "sophisticated" marketing techniques like bundling a soda with a burger. See the RAND Corporation's blog on obesity at http://www.rand.org/topics/obesity.html. For the paper on obesity's alleged growth, see Sturm, Roland and Hattori, Aiko, "Morbid Obesity Rates Continue to Rise Rapidly in the US", *International Journal of Obesity*, 2013, Vol. 37:6, pp. 889-891, http://www.ncbi.nlm.nih.gov/pmc/articles/PMC3527647/ DOI: 10.1038/ijo.2012.159.

[11] Cf. Olyslager, Femke and Conway, Lynn, "On the Calculation of the Prevalence of Transsexualism", 2007, paper presented at the WPATH 20th International Symposium in Chicago, http://ai.eecs.umich.edu/people/conway/TS/Prevalence/Reports/Prevalence%20of%20Transsexualism.pdf.

[12] Professional football players are likely to have ample muscle, whereas the BMI considers all excess weight to be fat. Still, the average weight of college and pro football players alike has increased substantially over the decades, and one scientist observes that, after reaching 114 kilograms (about 250 pounds), fat accumulation outpaces muscle and tends to be "distributed to the abdominal region." Cf. Bosch, Tyler A., et al, "Abdominal Body Composition Differences in NFL Football Players", *Journal of Strength & Conditioning Research*, 2014, Vol 28:12, pp. 3313-3319, Dec., DOI:10.1519/JSC.0000000000000650, and Anzel, A.R. *et al.*, "Changes in Height, Body Weight, and Body Composition in American Football Players from 1942 to 2011", *Journal of Strength and Conditioning Research*, 2013, Vol. 27:2, pp. 277-284, http://www.ncbi.nlm.nih.gov/pubmed/23222088, DOI: 10.1519/JSC.0b013e31827f4c08, and also Harp, Joyce B., *et al.*, "Obesity in the National Football League", *JAMA*, 2005, Vol. 293:9, pp. 1058 1062. http://jama.jamanetwork.com/article.aspx?articleid=200447, DOI: 10.1001/jama.293.9.1061-b.

[13] Cf. Leonard, William R., "The Global Diversity of Eating Patterns: Human Nutritional Health in Comparative Perspective", *Physiology & Behavior*, 2014, Vol. 134, pp. 5-14, http://www.ncbi.nlm.nih.gov/pubmed/24613505, DOI: 10.1016/j.physbeh.2014.02.050 and Cf. Marlow, FW and JC Berbesque, "Tubers as fallback foods and their impact on Hadza hunter-gatherers", American Journal of Physical Anthropology, 2009, Vol. 140:4, pp.751-758. DOI: 10.1002/ajpa.21040 http://onlinelibrary.wiley.com/doi/10.1002/ajpa.v140:4/issuetoc.

[14] A comprehensive review of extant data suggests the average life expectancy at birth among hunting and gathering groups with no access to modern medicine is 21 to 37 years. However, those who reach 45 have a further life expectancy of 14 to 24 years. Infant survival rates vary enormously between groups. Cf. Gurven, Michael and Kaplan, Hillard, "Longevity Among Hunter-Gatherers: A Cross-Cultural Examination", *Population and Development Review*, 2007, Vol. 33:2, pp. 321-365, http://onlinelibrary.wiley.com/doi/10.1111/j.1728-4457.2007.00171.x/abstract, DOI: 10.1111/j.1728-4457.2007.00171.x.

[15] Another contribution to the idea that the concept of an "obesity epidemic" is part of a salient cultural shift is from the sociologist Natalie Boero, who analyzed 751 articles published in *The New York Times* from 1990 to 2001 to track the emergence of "epidemic" as a descriptor. She concludes that the story is one of a "postmodern" epidemiology, in which "unevenly medicalized phenomena lacking a clear pathological basis get cast in the language and moral panic of 'traditional' epidemics." She suggests that obesity be construed as a social problem akin to that of teenage pregnancy, a biologically normal pattern changed by overriding social norms linked to status and plausible prospects, rather than tuberculosis, a classic infections disease. See her "All the News that's Fat to Print: The American 'Obesity Epidemic' and the Media", *Qualitative Sociology*, 2007, Vol. 30:1, pp. 41-60, http://link.springer.com/article/10.1007%2Fs11133-006-9010-4.

[16] The head of the Food and Agriculture Organization of the United Nations proposes that using food crops for fuel might lead to greater food production in some areas, noting

that the cost of gas in rural Africa can be three times the global average and thus discourages the use of tractors as well as the growth of processing and storage industries that would reduce agricultural losses and help eradicate local hunger. Cf. Graziano da Silva, José, "Food in the Age of Biofuels", Project Syndicate, June 25, 2015, http://www.project-syndicate.org/commentary/biofuels-food-security-climate-change-by-jose-graziano-da-silva-2015-06. For the WRI paper, see Searchinger, Tim and Heimlich, Ralph, "Avoiding Bioenergy Competition for Food Crops and Land", 2015, http://www.wri.org/sites/default/files/avoiding_bioenergy_competition_food_crops_land.pdf.

[17] "These findings suggest that news reports on the 'obesity epidemic' – and, by extension, on public health crises commonly blamed on personal behavior – may unintentionally activate prejudice", write Abigail Saguy, *et al.*, "Reporting Risk, Producing Prejudice: How News Reporting on Obesity Shapes Attitudes about Health Risk, Policy, and Prejudice", *Social Science & Medicine*, 2014, Vol. 111, pp. 125-133, http://www.ncbi.nlm.nih.gov/pubmed/24785268 DOI: 10.1016/j.socscimed.2014.03.026.

[18] The Smithsonian has excellent archival material from the trip, including the film. In his fine analysis of the trip, Joshua A. Bell wryly notes that the expedition was facilitated by a variety of colonial officials, missionaries, and even had a sizable escort of local constables, noting also that the personal papers of expedition leader E.W. Brandes, a pathologist working for the USDA, were destroyed by his wife, leaving only the images he shot along with an article and a book he wrote about his experience with a Neolithic world. Cf. his *Sugar Cane Hunting by Airplane: A Cinematic Narrative of Scientific Triumph and Discovery in the 'Remote Jungles'*, published in 2010 in *The Journal of Pacific History*, Vol. 45:1, pp. 37-56, DOI: 10.1080/00223344.2010.484166.

[19] Some linguistic scholars insist the Sanskrit word traces back to the Chinese term *Sha-Che*, literally the "Sand-Sugar plant." The term allegedly transformed phonetically into Sanskrit as *Sharkera*, the source of modern Hindi's *jaggery*, and went on to enter Arabic, where it became *Al-Sukker*, pronounced "Assuker." The Spanish word for sugar is *azucar*, while it is *zucchero* in Italian and *zucker* in German. Whatever the merits of the Chinese origin, the ancient Greeks already called it *sakkaron* in AD 56, passing to Latin as *saccharum*. Cf. Mahdihassan, S. "A Comparative Study of the Word Sugar and of its Equivalents in Hindustani as Traceable to Chinese", *American Journal of Chinese Medicine*, 1981, Vol. 9:3, pp. 187-192, http://www.ncbi.nlm.nih.gov/pubmed/6764089.

[20] Sugar cane's hyper-efficiency has intensified since humans began exploiting the plant and could even seem pathological! When the plant flowers, it emits very small pollens that have a half-life of only 12 minutes and are no longer viable after 35 minutes according to Australia's Gene Technology Regulator.

[21] Cerling's work was part of a battery of related research published in 2013. See Cerling, Thure, *et al.*, "Stable Isotope-based Diet Reconstructions of Turkana Basin Hominins", *PNAS*, 2013. Vol. 110:26, pp.10501-10506, DOI: 10.1073/pnas.1222568110. Cerling notes that isotopes don't reveal whether the teeth chewed C4 plants or animals that in turn ate the new kind of plants. He noted that herbivores in the Turkana Basin where he focused had mostly shifted to C4. Today, rhinos and giraffes are C3 eaters, zebras and warthogs C4 grazers, with some sticking to C3 plants, while impalas and gazelles, like hominids, ate both. Cerling's work was part of a series in the 2013 *Proceedings of the National Academy of Sciences* volume. In another, Matt Sponheimer notes the C4 dietary

change's likely role in encephalization of the brain, the emergence of bipedalism, and also the social and cultural practices of human groups in open landscapes compared to dense woodland. Two other papers in the series highlight how *Australopithecus anamensis*, a hominid species living 4 million years ago, rarely consumed C4 foods despite their presence, while *Paranthropus boisei*, living in the same region 2 million years later, obtained 80 percent of its diet from C4 sources. That's something that advocates of the "Paleolithic diet", who abhor C4 carbohydrates such as sugar and maize and prefer vegetables and meat, may wish to chew on!

[22] Cf. Richards, Michael *et al.*, "Isotopic Evidence of the Diets of European Neanderthals and Early Modern Humans", *PNAS*, 2009, Vol. 106:38, http://www.pnas.org/content/106/38/16034.full.pdf.

[23] He suggests that the evolution of C4 photosynthesis required the co-option of photosynthesis components, all originating from ancient bacteria, from other plants "into a new function and, in many cases, their adaptation for the novel metabolic context." Cf. Osborne, C. and Pascal-Antoine, Christine, "The Evolutionary Ecology of C4 Plants", *New Phytologist*, 2014, Vol 204:4, pp. 765-781, DOI:10.1111/nph.13033.

[24] Samuel Myers of the Harvard School of Public Health led a research team that subjected field sites in Japan, Australia, and the USA to atmospheric carbon dioxide levels predicted for the middle of this century. They found that C3 grains like wheat, barley, and rice, as well as legumes including field peas, showed drops in iron and protein levels of as much as 10 percent. Maize suffered a small decline and sorghum none. See his "Increasing CO2 Threatens Human Nutrition", *Nature*, 2014, Vol. 510, pp. 139-142, DOI: 10.1038/nature13179, http://www.nature.com/nature/journal/v510/n7503/full/nature13179.html.

[25] The IRRI's C4 rice project, funded by the Bill and Melinda Gates Foundation, started in 2008 with hopes to crack the code within twenty years. The IRRI has a long history of breeding rice varieties for higher output and particular climate conditions but says plant breeding seems to have exploited all the traits linked to high yield. C4 rice would be an anatomical innovation as the plant would have to be genetically tweaked to grow bundled sheath shells around its veins to store carbon dioxide. If successful, C4 rice would require less water and harness solar energy directly to grow food. Cf. Bullis, Kevin, "Supercharged Photosynthesis", *MIT Technology Review*, March 2015, http://irri-news.blogspot.it/2015/02/research-on-c4-rice-makes-mit.html.

[26] That acreage output was reported as the increase from the 2000-2005 period to the 2006-2011 period and is twice the scale of growth posted by Brazilian soybean. Cf. International Sugar Association, *Outlook of Sugar and Ethanol Production in Brazil*, 2012.

[27] Researchers in Nigeria found that applying nitrogen could limit the number of canes that flower to 2 percent, compared to 80 percent without the application that yielded 40 to 60 percent more than flowering types, although the base varieties in their comparison were not identical. See El Manhaly, M.A., *et al.*, "Control of Flowering in Two Commercial Sugar-cane Varieties", *Journal of Agricultural Sciences*, 1984, Vol. 103, pp. 333-338, https://www.unilorin.edu.ng/publications/abayomiya/Control%20of%20Flowering%20in%20Two%20Commerial%20Sugar-Cane%20Varaibles.pdf.

[28] Matt Ridley, in "Can Rice Match Maize's Yield?" published July 7, 2012 in the *Wall Street Journal*, noted that fourteen of the eighteen most pestilential weeds for farmers

are C4 plants. He also cited a real-time experiment on a farm run by the Institute of Soil Science in Nanjing, in which rice and barnyard grass, its enemy and a C4 plant, grew side by side in plots with normal conditions and again with the ambient level of carbon dioxide doubled. The rice yield was 38 percent higher by yield and the barnyard grass reduced by 47.9 percent, "because the vigorous rice shaded out the weeds." Here's the report on that: Zeng, Qing, "Elevated CO2 Effects on Nutrient Competition Between a C3 Crop and a C4 Weed", *Nutrient Cycling in Agroecosystems*, 2011, Vol. 89:1, pp. 93-104, http://link.springer.com/article/10.1007%2Fs10705-010-9379-z, DOI: 10.1007/s10705-010-9379-z.

29 The most assiduous modern interpreter of this relatively undiscussed ecological dimension of Marx's thought is University of Oregon professor John Bellamy Foster. See his "Marx and the Rift in the Universal Metabolism of Nature", *Monthly Review*, 2013, Vol. 65:7, http://monthlyreview.org/2013/12/01/marx-rift-universal-metabolism-nature/.

30 A superb review of the state of the art can be found in van der Weijde, Tim, *et al.*, "The Potential of C4 Grasses for Cellulosic Biofuel Production", *Frontiers in Plant Science*, 2013, Vol. 4, http://www.ncbi.nlm.nih.gov/pmc/articles/PMC3642498/#B67, DOI:10.3389/fpls.2013.00107. The authors note that there are potentially 1.5 billion tonnes of available biomass from current agricultural production of sugar cane, maize, and sorghum alone. They are all C4 crops, as are eleven of the world's twelve most productive crops. While they note that sugar cane ethanol has birthed an active breeding effort aimed at higher yield, even at the cost of low-sucrose yield, they contest the assumption that the plant must make a biological tradeoff between sucrose and biomass volume. They also suggest that while Europeans appear opposed to genetic modification of foods, they are likely to loosen their policy opposition for biofuel plants. Dual-use versions could prove thorny in that regard.

31 The precise role of fish is a bit of a mystery. Many historical accounts suggest fish was seen as a poor food source, but many also suggest that elites ate it anyway. Fish consumption can leave carbon traces in bone collagen that confound C4 counts, although their higher nitrogen component can eventually also be assessed. Cf. Tafuri, Mary Anne, "Stable Isotope Evidence for the Consumption of Millet and Other Plants in Bronze Age Italy", *American Journal of Physical Anthropology*, 2009, Vol. 139:2, pp. 146-153, http://onlinelibrary.wiley.com/doi/10.1002/ajpa.20955/abstract;jsessionid=81470119DAFF8EF53D3EF2AC2F54F57B.f04t03, DOI: 10.1002/ajpa.20955. For Croatia, see Lightfood, E., *et al.*, "Changing Cultures, Changing Cuisines: Cultural Transitions and Dietary Change in Iron Age, Roman and Early Medieval Croatia", *American Journal of Physical Anthropology*, 2012, Vol. 148:4, pp. 543-556, http://www.ncbi.nlm.nih.gov/pubmed/22552855, DOI 10.1002/adjpa.22070,.

32 Gandia's sugar exports spurred a confectionery craze in Barcelona, home to one of the earliest cookbooks devoted to sweets in Europe, the fifteenth-century *Llibre de totes maneres de confits*. Michelle Alexander of the University of York led the isotope study. Cf. "Diet, Society and Economy in Late Medieval Spain: Stable Isotope Evidence from Muslims and Christians from Gandia, Valencia", *American Journal of Physical Anthropology*, 2015, Vol. 156:2, pp. 263-273, http://www.ncbi.nlm.nih.gov/pubmed/25351146/, DOI: 10.1002/ajpa.22647.

33 Similar isotope research on Ibiza, which was ruled by Carthage, then Byzantium and then al-Andalus, used bones spanning 3,500 years. The sampling techniques also evi-

denced significant social mobility as a number of the skeletons were identified as immigrants to the island. The last samples, during the Islamic era, were the only to show substantial C4 traces. Cf. Fuller, B.T., "Investigation of Diachronic Dietary Patterns on the Islands of Ibiza and Formentera", *American Journal of Physical Anthropology*, 2012, Vol. 143:4, pp. 512-522, http://onlinelibrary.wiley.com/enhanced/doi/10.1002/ajpa.21334/.

[34] Avicenna, the Persian scholar said to have memorized Aristotle by the age of 15, also used the taste test and the honey/urine analogy. His book *The Canon of Medicine* was available in translation in Italy in the late 1400s and may have been the indirect source for Willis. Garabed Eknoyan and Judit Nagy offer a comprehensive account extending up to the early 1900s in "A History of Diabetes Mellitus or How a Disease of the Kidneys Evolved into a Kidney Disease", *Advances in Chronic Kidney Disease*, 2005, Vol. 12:2, pp. 223-229, http://www.ackdjournal.org/article/S1548-5595(05)00026-1/fulltext, DOI: doi.org/10.1053/j.ackd.2005.01.002.

[35] Sidney Mintz's *Sweetness and Power: The Place of Sugar in Modern History*, Penguin Books, 1986 is a superb and famous work with a deep geopolitical focus on an industry that moved millions of people around the world. Mintz has done extensive work on the anthropology of food, much of it focusing on what he calls "tropical drugs" such as sugar and coffee – a drink, he notes, that is not taken with sugar in its original home.

[36] Wages would later rise as large-scale coal extraction lowered energy prices, but the big jump didn't happen until the second half of the nineteenth century. The wage data come from Allen, Robert C., "Why Was the Industrial Revolution British?", *VoxEU*, May 15, 2009, http://www.voxeu.org/article/why-was-industrial-revolution-british.

[37] Hogarth was apparently no friend of Mediterranean diet types. He was a founding member of the Sublime Society of Beefsteaks and his oil painting *The Gate of Calais* exudes xenophobia with its depiction of a scrawny French soldier, starving Scottish refugees and a fat Catholic monk. In what some might see as Protestant extremism, he also made a set of prints contrasting the fates of a committed and a wayward apprentice in the trades. Two other series, *A Harlot's Progress* and *The Rake's Progress*, depict bad endings for a country lass who comes to the city and ends up a prostitute who dies young, and a wealthy heir who fritters away his money and ends up in a madhouse. Despite such unrelenting insistence on individual responsibility, he has been evoked in today's public health discourse as in fact sympathetic to the working poor. Cf. Muldoon, Sascha, "Hogarth's 'Gin Lane' and 'Bear Street'", *International Journal of Surgery*, 2005, Vol. 3:2, pp. 159-162, http://www.sciencedirect.com/science/article/pii/S174391910500004X?np=y, DOI: 10.1016/j.ijsu.2005.03.006.

[38] The text can be read in full at The Internet Archive, a San Francisco-based nonprofit digitizing service of historical documents for public access. See https://archive.org/stream/anenquiryintoca00fielgoog#page/n42/mode/2up.

[39] Abel, Ernest L., "The Gin Epidemic: Much Ado About What?" *Alcohol and Alcoholism*, 2001, Vol. 36:5, pp. 401-405, DOI: org/10.1093/alcalc/36.5.401, http://alcalc.oxfordjournals.org/content/36/5/401.

[40] Alcohol, and usually for the most part beer, contributed three times more calorie intake in the eighteenth and nineteenth centuries than in 1975, according to nutrition experts at the UK's Ministry of Agriculture. Spring, J. A. and Buss, David H., "Three Cen-

turies of Alcohol in the British Diet",, *Nature*, 1977, Vol. 270, pp. 567-572, http://www.nature.com/nature/journal/v270/n5638/abs/270567a0.html, DOI: 10.1038/270567a0.

[41] Kayleigh Marie DePriest uncovered this document, which laments the frequent drunken state of beggars and children of both sexes, rending them "unfit for labour." See her "The 'Gin Epidemic': London's Public Health Crisis", *Legacy*, 2009, Vol. 9, http://www.earlymodernengland.com/2012/09/the-gin-epidemic-londons-public-health-crisis/.

[42] Holden also worried that barley growers would go bust without a client base for the spirit their product made. See his "The trial of the spirits, or, Some considerations upon the pernicious consequences of the gin-trade to Great Britain", London, T. Cooper, 1736. For the gin advocate, see T.S., "A Proper Reply to a Scandalous Libel,... the Trial of the Spirits", London, J. Roberts, 1736, http://www.worldcat.org/title/proper-reply-to-a-scandalous-libel-intituled-the-trial-of-the-spirits-in-a-letter-to-the-author/oclc/642667625.

[43] Cf. Aaron, Paul and Musto, David, "Temperance and Prohibition in America", a 1981 paper commissioned by the US National Research Council on Alternative Policies Affecting the Prevention of Alcohol Abuse and Alcoholism, http://www.ncbi.nlm.nih.gov/books/NBK216414/?report=reader#_NBK216414_pubdet_.

[44] Dermota, Petra, *et al.*, "Health Literacy and Substance Abuse in Young Swiss Men", *International Journal of Public Health*, 2013, Vol. 58:6, pp. 939-948, http://link.springer.com/article/10.1007%2Fs00038-013-0487-9#page-1.

[45] Finkelstein's hypothetical 26 percent average tax on sugary drinks is in fact based on half a US penny per ounce, which is half the levy proposed by former New York City mayor, Michael Bloomberg. The 2013 study can be consulted at Finkelstein, Eric, *et al.*, "Implications of a Sugar-sweetened Beverage (SSB) Tax when Substitutions to Non-beverage Items are Considered", *Journal of Health Economics*, 2013, Vol. 32:1, pp. 219-239, http://www.ncbi.nlm.nih.gov/pubmed/23202266, DOI: 10.1016/j.jhealeco.2012.10.005, while the more elaborate model used in 2014, which finds that lower-income families would actually face larger welfare reductions in absolute terms than higher-income households is explained in Zhen, C., *et al.*, "Predicting the Effects of Sugar-sweetened Beverage Taxes on Food and Beverage Demand in a Large Demand System", *American Journal of Agricultural Economics*, 2014, Vol. 96:1, pp. 1-25, http://www.ncbi.nlm.nih.gov/pmc/articles/PMC4022288/, DOI: 10.1093/ajae/aat049. The *Take Care New York 2012* report can be found at http://www.nyc.gov/html/doh/downloads/pdf/tcny/tcny-2012.pdf.

[46] In a randomized clinical trial designed to test weight-loss effects exclusively from cutting back on caloric beverages, including alcohol, juice and coffee and tea if taken with sugar, adults in North Carolina with average BMIs of 36 agreed to drink non-caloric beverages for six months. Cutting back the equivalent of two cans of soda a day led to shedding 2 kilograms, an outcome only 25 percent as large as touted by the New York advertising firm. Cf. Tate, Deborah F., "Replacing Caloric Beverages with Water or Diet Beverages for Weight Loss in Adults", *American Journal of Clinical Nutrition*, 2012, Vol. 95:3, pp. 555-563, http://www.ncbi.nlm.nih.gov/pmc/articles/PMC3632875/, DOI: 10.3945/ajcn.111.026278.

Chapter 3

1 The data, which does not include high-fructose corn syrup widely used for soft drinks in the USA, comes from Paris-based Sucres & Denrées, a company that ships and distributes 10 percent of the world's sugar. It estimates 180 million tonnes are produced and 90 million consumed; the rest have industrial uses including ethanol. Only 49 million tonnes are traded across borders, reflecting the importance countries have given to producing it domestically, which is now done in 120 nations. See http://www.sucden.com/.

2 "Timely, dramatic, and effective development and implementation of corrective programs/policies are needed to avoid the otherwise inevitable health and societal consequences implied by our projections", writes Youfa Wang and colleagues, adding that theirs is probably a conservative estimate. Cf. "Will All Americans Become Overweight or Obese? Estimating the Progression and Cost of the US Obesity Epidemic", *Obesity*, 2008, Vol. 16, pp. 2323-2330, http://www.ncbi.nlm.nih.gov/pubmed/18719634, DOI:10.1038/oby.2008.351.

3 The authors use a complex formula for their calculations. They also say that obesity has driven the lifetime risk of diabetes among people in the USA up to between 30 and 40 percent and add that diabetes typically shortens lives by thirteen years. Cf. Olshanksy, S. Jay, et al, "A Potential Decline in Life Expectancy in the United States in the 21st Century", *New England Journal of Medicine*, 2005, Vol. 352, pp. 1138-1145, http://www.nejm.org/doi/full/10.1056/NEJMsr043743#t=articleTop, DOI: 10.1056/NEJMsr043743.

4 The Sanskrit text, one of the world's all-time literary bestsellers, was adapted for modern use by Jared Diamond in his popular thesis that the invention of agriculture was "the worst mistake in the history of the human race", introducing health problems, social inequality, and despotism. He published a short version of his view in 1999 in the magazine *Discover*. Cf. http://discovermagazine.com/1987/may/02-the-worst-mistake-in-the-history-of-the-human-race.

5 Cf. Basu, Sanjay, *et al.*, "Diabetes Prevalence: An Econometric Analysis of Repeated Cross-Sectional Data", *Plos*, 2013, http://journals.plos.org/plosone/article?id=10.1371/journal.pone.0057873, DOI: 0.1371/journale.pone.0057873.

6 A fascinating tour de force full of striking details, the argument suggests that the "underlying drivers of consumption" of such unhealthy commodities lie in supply-side factors such as free trade agreements and market dominance by global brands rather than in any demand-side factors that might propel citizens caught up in stressful social changes to seek out high-energy foods. Cf. Stuckler, David, *et al.*, "Manufacturing Epidemics: The Role of Global Producers in Increased Consumption of Unhealthy Commodities Including Processed Foods, Alcohol and Tobacco", *Plos Medicine*, 2012, Vol. 9:6, http://www.ncbi.nlm.nih.gov/pmc/articles/PMC3383750/, DOI: 10.1371/journal.pmed.1001235.

7 The prevalence of metabolic syndrome was 41 percent for Finnish men aged 45 to 64 educated through the ninth grade, compared to 21 percent for those who had a university degree; for women, the rates were 27 and 14 percent respectively. No less than 78 percent of the men surveyed, randomly and from across the country, qualified as obese

under the WHO definition of a BMI above 30. Cf. Silventoinen, Karri, *et al.*, "Educational Inequalities in the Metabolic Syndrome and Coronary Heart Disease Among Middle-aged Men and Women", *International Journal of Epidemiology*, 2005, Vol. 4:2, pp.327-334, http://ije.oxfordjournals.org/content/34/2/327.full, DOI: 10.1093/ije/dyi007.

8 The civil servants canvassed were part of the Whitehall II sample. An earlier long-term survey of British civil servants found there was algorithmic regularity to a pattern whereby at every level of the hierarchy a junior employee was more likely to develop a chronic disease than his or her senior manager. Cf. Chandola, Tarani *et al.*, "Chronic stress at work and the metabolic syndrome: prospective study", *BMJ*, 2006, Vol. 332, pp. 521-525 http://www.ncbi.nlm.nih.gov/pmc/articles/PMC1388129. DOI: 10.1136/dmj.38693.435301.80

9 Asked specifically about the state of food and agriculture, twice as many said things are getting worse as those who said they are getting better. One of Lusk's sounding points is that taxing cheaper sugary and fatty foods to subsidize vegetables is likely to end up as a fiscal subsidy of the affluent by the poor. Cf. http://jaysonlusk.com/blog/2015/7/14/food-demand-survey-foods-july-2015.

10 The US FDA says four times the amount of antibiotics given to people are fed to animals in sub-therapeutic doses designed to stoke weight gain. The technique was discovered in 1946, six years before the McDonald brothers commissioned their first set of golden arches. Cf. Riley, Lee W., "Obesity in the United States – Dysbiosis from Exposure to Low-Dose Antibiotics?" *Frontiers of Public Health*, 2013, Vol.1, http://www.ncbi.nlm.nih.gov/pmc/articles/PMC3867737/, DOI:10.3389/fpubh.2013.00069.

11 The series begins here: Gornall, Jonathan, "Sugar: Spinning a Web of Influence", *BMJ*, 2015, Vol. 350, http://www.bmj.com/content/350/bmj.h231, DOI: 10.1136/bmj.h231.

12 Dietary supplement companies are hoping the anti-obesity campaign will increase popular usage of the term "blood sugar" and in turn trigger demand for products claiming to manage blood glucose. "Anything which could make formerly off-limits food permissible has great potential", Jeff Hilton, founder of one marketing and branding expert told The Food Navigator Cf. Daniells, Stephen, "Pharmachem: The Potential Market for Products Addressing Excess Sugar Consumption is Huge, Oct. 29, 2013, http://www.foodnavigator-usa.com/Suppliers2/Pharmachem-The-potential-market-for-products-addressing-excess-sugar-consumption-is-huge.

13 As reported by Colby Vorland while blogging the American Society for Nutrition's annual assembly. Cf. https://www.nutrition.org/asn-blog/2014/04/addressing-the-bias-in-nutrition-science/.

14 It may be that lobby-funded research is less biased due to different kinds of "actionable results". It is widely assumed that businesses seek profit while public officials seek to muster support for re-appointment or election. Cf. Cope, Mark B. and Allison, David B., "White Hat Bias: A Threat to the Integrity of Scientific Reporting", *Acta Paediatrica*, 2010, Vol. 99:11, pp.1615-1617, http://onlinelibrary.wiley.com/doi/10.1111/j.1651-2227.2010.02006.x/full, DOI: 10.1111/j.1651-2227.2010.02006.x, and Cope, Mark B. and Allison, David B., "White Hat Bias: Examples of its Presence in Obesity Research and a Call for Renewed Commitment to Faithfulness in Research Reporting", *International Journal of Obesity*, 2010, Vol. 34:1, http://www.ncbi.nlm.nih.gov/pmc/articles/PMC2815336/, DOI: 10.1038/ijo.2009.239.

[15] Cf. Behan, Donald B. and Cox, Samuel H., "Obesity and its Relation to Morbidity and Obesity Costs", Society of Actuaries, Committee on Life Insurance Research, 2010, https://www.soa.org/research/research-projects/life-insurance/research-obesity-relation-mortality.aspx.

[16] The WHO also has a new study saying that household energy use in developing nations, often using kerosene stoves, causes 3.5 million deaths a year. Cf. Williams, Kendra N., *et al.*, "Health Impacts of Household Energy Use: Indicators of Exposure to Air Pollution and Other Risks", *WHO Bulletin*, 2015, Vol. 93:7, pp. 437-512, http://www.who.int/bulletin/volumes/93/7/14-144923/en/, DOI:10.2471/BLT.14.144923. For the European study, see "Economic Cost of the Health Impact of Air Pollution in Europe", WHO, 2015, http://www.euro.who.int/en/media-centre/events/events/2015/04/ehp-mid-term-review/publications/economic-cost-of-the-health-impact-of-air-pollution-in-europe. For tax rates on income, excluding social security charges which are for retirement schemes, see the Organization for Economic Cooperation and Development, http://www.oecd-ilibrary.org/taxation/taxes-on-personal-income_20758510-table4.

[17] If passed, registered dietitians and nutrition professionals as well as many "community-based lifestyle counseling programs" will be able to prescribe reimbursable treatment programs. Here's the text of the bill: https://www.govtrack.us/congress/bills/114/hr2404/text.

[18] Almost half the subjects in the *JAMA* experiment had a BMI below 35. Cf. Courcoulas, Anita P., *et al.*, "Three-Year Outcomes of Bariatric Surgery vs Lifestyle Intervention for Type 2 Diabetes Treatment", *JAMA Surgery*, 2015, http://archsurg.jamanetwork.com/article.aspx?articleid=2362353, DOI: 10.1001/jamasurg.2015.1534.

[19] Cremieux is positive that the societal burdens linked to the swelling ranks of the obese will soon lead policy-makers in the USA, Canada, France, China, and Brazil to warm to the pharmaceutical industry's cause. Somewhat amazingly he says there is "limited real world information available" for insurance payers to make decisions regarding weight policy, revealing that he is frustrated by bias in the reams of data actually published on the subject. The new drugs are lorcaserin, phentermine/topiramate extended release, naltrexone/bupropion extended release, and liraglutide. Cf. Frois, Christian and Cremieux, Pierre-Yves, "For a Step Change to Curb the Obesity Epidemic", *PharmacoEconomics*, 2015, Vol. 33, pp. 613-617, http://link.springer.com/article/10.1007/s40273-015-0303-x, DOI: 10.1007/s40273-015-0303-x.

[20] Pharmaceutical companies complain that regulatory approval for anti-obesity drugs is hard to obtain the USA because the US FDA now wants to see the results of a long-term cardiovascular outcome trials in the application phase. Cf. Baum, Charles, *et al.*, "The Challenges and Opportunities Associated with Reimbursement for Obesity Pharmacotherapy in the USA", *PharmacoEconomics*, 2015, Vol. 33, pp. 643-653, http://link.springer.com/article/10.1007/s40273-015-0264-0/fulltext.html, DOI: 10.1007/s40273-015-0264-0.

[21] In an accomplished multipronged media barrage, Analysis Group published its findings with a report, a paper in the *Journal of Clinical Psychiatry* and a guest blog on *Scientific American*'s website. Paul E. Greenberg said that the overall societal cost of depression – treated with drugs such as Prozac or Zoloft – had risen only slightly in the past twenty years despite many more people receiving treatment, which he saw not as proof of ef-

fectiveness but rather as that "the quality of ... treatment was generally not very good." Cf. "The Growing Economic Burden of Depression in the U.S.", *Scientific American*, Feb. 25, 2015, http://blogs.scientificamerican.com/mind-guest-blog/the-growing-economic-burden-of-depression-in-the-u-s/. By way of comparison, the American Diabetes Association estimates that the total economic burden of diabetes in the USA in 2012, two years later than the reference year for the depression analysis, was $245 billion. Cf. "Economic Costs of Diabetes in the U.S. in 2012", *Diabetes Care*, 2013, Vol. 36:4, http://care.diabetesjournals.org/content/36/4/1033.ful, DOI: 10.2337/dc12-2625.

22 It has long been assumed that statins may numb insulin sensitivity, but the Finnish study used the largest data sample to date and found the largest impact. To be clear, over the six years, 11.2 percent of the people treated with statins developed diabetes compared to 58 percent of those who did not. Cf. Cederberg, Henna, *et al.*, "Increased risk of diabetes with statin treatment is associated with impaired insulin sensitivity and insulin secretion: a 6-year Follow-up Study of the METSIM Cohort", *Diabetologia*, 2015, Vol. 58:5, pp. 1109-1117, http://www.ncbi.nlm.nih.gov/pubmed/25754552, DOI 10.1007/s00125-015-3528-5. Cederberg emphasized that the research did not mean statins were ineffective, but that many patients may have to make a choice. One medical professional reacted by saying "this study did not examine the benefits of statin therapy, it examined only the risk of diabetes." For the headline, see http://www.pharmaceutical-journal.com/news-and-analysis/research-briefing/finnish-study-explores-association-between-statin-use-and-diabetes/20068110.article.

23 Somewhat surprisingly for a person so associated with obesity, his 3 percent argument is made on the base of dental caries in a study that relies primarily on Japanese wartime data. Cf. Sheiham, Aubrey and James, W. Philip T., "A Reappraisal of the Quantitative Relationship Between Sugar Intake and Dental Caries: The Need for New Criteria for Developing Goals for Sugar Intake", *BMC Public Health*, 2014, Vol. 14, http://www.biomedcentral.com/1471-2458/14/863, DOI: 10.1186/1471-2458-14-863.

24 James notes that an extra 10 kilograms of weight will likely require a permanent extra daily intake of 200 or 300 calories. Then, in a refreshingly skeptical flourish, he notes that "one is fortunate if one can be confident of measuring energy intake to within 500 kilocalories a day of the true figure." Cf. "The Epidemiology of Obesity: The Size of the Problem", *Journal of Internal Medicine*, 2008, Vol. 263, pp. 336-352, http://www.researchgate.net/publication/5540632_The_epidemiology_of_obesity_The_size_of_the_problem, DOI: 10.1111/j.1365-2796.2008.01922.x.

25 Cf. Young, Edwin and Scott Kantor, Linda, "Moving Toward the Food Guide Pyramid: Implications for U.S. Agriculture", *USDA*, 1999, Agricultural Economic Report No. 779, http://www.ers.usda.gov/publications/aer-agricultural-economic-report/aer779.aspx.

26 Thallium has the toxicity of cadmium or mercury. Cf. Oppenheimer, Todd, "The Vegetable Detective", *Craftsmanship*, 2015, http://craftsmanship.net/the-vegetable-detective/. Researchers in New Zealand tested eleven plants for their ability to transport the toxin. At just 0.7 milligrams of thallium for each kilogram of soil they found spinach, watercress, turnip, and radish could not be safely eaten although tomatoes, onions, and lettuce didn't absorb the traces. They suggested that contaminated fields could be mined for the chemical – currently produced only in Macedonia – while they leeched it out of the soil, a process that could take up to thirty years. Writing in 2001, they

also mentioned thallium had been extensively found at produce markets in France and also in rapeseed, a relative of kale and the core element of a cooking oil making inroads in European restaurants today. Cf. LaCoste, Cheer, *et al.*, "Uptake of Thallium by Vegetables: Its Significance for Human Health, Phytoremediation, and Phytomining", *Journal of Plant Nutrition*, 2001, Vol. 24:8, pp. 1205-1215, http://www.kiwiscience.com/JournalArticles/JPlantNutrition2001.pdf.

27 Bellemare likes the growth in farmers' markets but simply notes that minimally processed vegetables "provide new ecosystems within which pathogens can emerge and evolve" and that farmers' markets are by nature less subject to controls. Food-borne illnesses cause 1,400 deaths, 55,000 hospitalizations and cost $51 billion annually in the USA alone, he adds. Cf. Bellemare, Marc F., et al, "Farmers Markets and Food-Borne Illnesses", 2015, http://marcfbellemare.com/wordpress/wp-content/uploads/2015/07/BellemareKingNguyenFarmersMarketsJuly2015.pdf, *Campylobacter jejuni* is a street-fighting bug which in small numbers can colonize the human gut and bully indigenous microbes. Despite the fact that its genome has been sequenced just how it does so is a mystery. Scientists are flummoxed by its extreme metabolic flexibility as it doesn't seem to use glucose or carbohydrates for energy. Serious infections can lead to human immune systems attacking the body's own nerves, resulting in paralysis and the need for intensive medical care. Cf. Stahl, Martin *et al.*, "Nutrient Acquisition and Metabolism by Campylobacter jejuni", *Frontiers in Cellular and Infection Microbiology*, 2012, Vol.2:5 http://www.ncbi.nlm.nih.gov/pmc/articles/PMC3417520/.DOI: 10.3389/fcimb.2012.00005

28 A closer reading of the BMI trend, such as it is, casts doubt on the official view that there is a recent obesity epidemic. John Komlos and Marek Brabec reviewed historical data, including archives showing that the average BMI for a 19-year-old cadet at the West Point Military Academy – not exactly an institution for the poor – was 20.5 in the nineteenth century. The two big surges correlate strikingly with the introduction of the automobile and the television. The authors also note that the big changes have occurred among the heaviest tenth of the population, who now weigh 128 pounds more than in 1900, a gain eleven times greater than the slimmest tenth. Cf. "The Evolution of BMI Values of US Adults: 1882-1987", August 2010, http://www.voxeu.org/article/100-years-us-obesity.

29 The Mediterranean Basin has the highest output compared to domestic need in the world, explaining the traditional dietary virtues of the region, although today fruit and vegetable output is often exported, often as juice, reducing its domestic availability. Montenegro is the world champion in fibrous virtue, producing more than twice as many fruit and vegetables as it needs. Unfortunately, the Balkan country is half the size of Vermont. Interestingly, China, the world's most populous country, has a very hefty fruit and vegetable surplus. The authors used data on a nation-by-nation basis and note that transportation limitations mean access to fruit and vegetables may be lower than reported in some urban centers. See Siegel, Karen R., *et al.*, "Do We Produce Enough Fruits and Vegetables to Meet Global Health Need?" *Plos*, 2014, http://journals.plos.org/plosone/article?id=10.1371/journal.pone.0104059, DOI: 10.1371/journal.pone.0104059.

30 One of the first and most famous animal experiments was in fact done with dogs. In 1816, François Magendie described how a three-year-old dog died after 32 days during

which he fed it only sugar. Magendie, who established that rabies could be transmitted but long rejected the idea that cholera was contagious, was an avid experimentalist, earning a caricature in Balzac as a skeptic "who believed only in the scalpel." He had once held that "dogs can live very well on bread alone" but when he tested that, the dog lasted only fifty days. He also tried feeding dogs just olive oil, gum, and butter, with the same result. In the end he decided that "diversity and multiplicity of aliments is an important rule of hygiene." The experiments were done under the aegis of a public commission to determine whether hospitals might save money by serving boiled bones instead of meat. Cf. Carpenter, Kenneth J., "A Short History of Nutritional Science", *Journal of Nutrition*, 2003, Vol. 133:3, pp. 638-645, http://jn.nutrition.org/content/133/3/638.full.

31 It turns out that the fruit fly will become obese if you give it a high-sugar diet in it's the larval stage, when literally all the flies do is eat continuously. Infant *Drosophila melanogaster* were given a diet with excess dietary sugars but not extra fats or proteins, and quickly showed signs of insulin resistance. These larvae were given a diet consisting of six times more sucrose than their normal peers and more than 86 percent of their calories as carbohydrates. They were smaller than usual and spent up to twice the usual five days to turn into adult flies, traits shared by peers fed high-fat and high-protein diets. Cf. Musselman, Laura Palanker, "A High-sugar Diet Produces Obesity and Insulin Resistance in Wild-type Drosophila", *Disease Models and Mechanisms*, 2011, Vol. 4:6, pp. 842-849, http://www.ncbi.nlm.nih.gov/pmc/articles/PMC3209653/, DOI: 10.1242/dmm.007948.

32 Some 70 percent of the rats on the high-fat diet succeeded in becoming obese, but the researchers were palpably keen to produce fat rats more quickly and suggested that forced feeding should replace the ad libitum regime. The rate for those on the "best" diet comprising mostly sucrose was far lower but the researchers noted that a "small percentage" of them went through a belated growth "spurt" that led them close to the one-kilogram target at the age of one year. Intriguingly the authors suggested that a form of accelerated metabolic ageing might be taking place in those cases. Cf. Mickelsen, Olaf, *et al.*, "Production of Obesity in Rats by Feeding High-Fat Diets", *Experimental Obesity, Journal of Nutrition*, 1955, http://jn.nutrition.org/content/57/4/541.full.pdf.

33 Hatori, Megumi *et al.*, "Time-Restricted Feeding Without Reducing Caloric Intake Prevents Metabolic Diseases in Mice Fed a High-Fat Diet", *Cell Metabolism*, 2012, Vol. 15:6, pp. 848-860, http://www.sciencedirect.com/science/article/pii/S1550413112001891, DOI:10.1016/j.cmet.2012.04.019.

34 Sleep deprivation lowers leptin levels, which are a signal of fullness and suppress appetites, while raising levels of ghrelin, which is engaged in weight regulation that in simple terms signals hunger; it is also released when the stomach is empty. Cf. Patel, Sanjay R., *et al.*, "Association Between Reduced Sleep and Weight Gain in Women", *American Journal of Epidemiology*, 2006, Vol. 164:10, pp. 947-954, http://www.ncbi.nlm.nih.gov/pmc/articles/PMC3496783/, DOI: 10.1093/aje/kwj280. Sleep isn't just an American problem. A study of New Zealanders with regular jobs found that those with "social jetlag", in which people's internal "social clocks" clashed with their circadian rhythms, tended to have higher BMI and metabolic dysfunction, suggesting that work schedules might often be a "policy and practice" fostering obesity and diabetes. Cf. Parsons, M.J.,

et al., "Social Jetlag, Obesity and Metabolic disorder: Investigation in a Cohort Study", *International Journal of Obesity*, 2014, http://www.nature.com/ijo/journal/v39/n5/full/ijo2014201a.html, DOI: 10.1038/ijo.2014.201.

[35] Hoch, Tobias *et al.*, "Snack food intake in ad libitum fed rats is triggered by the combination of fat and carbohydrates", *Frontiers of Psychology*, 2014, Vol. 5 http://www.ncbi.nlm.nih.gov/pmc/articles/PMC3978285/. DOI: 10.3389//fpsyg.2014.00250

[36] The authors allow that sugar-eating rats might become obese over the long run. Cf. La Fleur, S.E., *et al.*, "A Free-choice High-fat, High-sugar Diet Induces Changes in Arcuate Neuropeptide Expression that Support Hyperphagia", *International Journal of Obesity*, 2010, Vol. 34, pp. 537-546, http://www.nature.com/ijo/journal/v34/n3/full/ijo2009257a.html, DOI:10.1038/ijo.2009.257.

[37] The pythons were treated to portions equal to one-fourth of their body weight and conked out for two weeks after eating them. Cf. Boback, S.M., *et al.*, "Cooking and Grinding Reduces the Cost of Meat Digestion", *Comparative Biochemistry and Physiology*, 2007, Vol. 148:3, pp. 651-656, http://www.ncbi.nlm.nih.gov/pubmed/17827047, DOI: 10.1016/j.cbpa.2007.08.014.

[38] Nutritional balance is in fact almost always the product of combinations of foods rather than single elements, according to fascinating analyses of more than 1,000 raw food types being done by a Korean research team. For the record, purists seeking maximal nutritional fitness in a single food should, according to this analysis, eat almonds, ocean perch, and cherimoya, a creamy-fleshed fruit originating in South America and now grown in warm climates around the world, also known as the "custard apple" and described by Mark Twain as "the most delicious fruit known to men." Cf. Kim, Seunghyeon, *et al.*, "Uncovering the Nutritional Landscape of Food", *Plos*, 2015, http://journals.plos.org/plosone/article?id=10.1371/journal.pone.0118697, DOI: 10.1371/journal.pone.0118697. Garlic mustard is also drawing new attention as an immunity-boosting and cholesterol-chopping plant that was eaten from the Mesolithic era through the mid-1800s but is now decried as an invasive plant. It is, for the record, not related to garlic, and hence has nothing to do with the recent commercial boom in "aioli garlic mustard sauce."

[39] Fructose increased iron-induced ferritin formation in key cells by up to 300 percent. This was also true for HFCS, although the authors note that it can be negated if consumed as cola, which contains caffeine, a polyphenol known to decrease the absorption of non-heme iron, the kind vegetables provide. Of course, excess iron poses a major health problem, but iron deficiency causes anemia, low birth weight and can impair cognitive development. Cf. Christides, Tatiana and Sharp, Paul, "Sugars Increase Non-Heme Iron Bioavailability in Human Epithelial Intestinal and Liver Cells", *Plos*, 2013, http://journals.plos.org/plosone/article?id=10.1371/journal.pone.0083031, DOI: 10.1371/journal.pone.0083031.

[40] Cf. Young, Nicholas A., et al, "Oral Administration of Nano-Emulsion Curcumin in Mice Suppresses Inflammatory-Induced NFkB Signaling and Macrophage Migration", *Plos*, 2014, http://journals.plos.org/plosone/article?id=10.1371/journal.pone.0111559, DOI: 10.1371/journal.pone.0111559.

[41] The cultural aspects of dietary patterns are hard to fathom but can never be underestimated. In a brilliant big data-crunching exercise based on more than 50,000 traditional

recipes, researchers in India found there is a large East-West gap in food preferences, with westerners and especially North Americans liking so-called "positive food pairing" involving mixing ingredients that share flavour compounds to enhance palatability – think creamy French sauce – while the Asian penchant is to use spices to create "negative food pairing" – think garlic with sesame – which they interpret as reflecting traditional interest in medicinal foods and diets. Interestingly, the authors found that Southern European food patterns show some tendency towards negative pairing, suggesting a historic role for quasi-medicinal plants. For the study and brilliant graphics, cf. Ahn, Yog-Yeol, *et al.*, "Flavor Network and the Principles of Food Pairing", *Scientific Reports*, 2011, http://www.nature.com/srep/2011/111215/srep00196/full/srep00196.html, DOI: 10.1038/srep00196. Anupam Jain and colleagues used a similar analysis for Indian food, see "Spices Form the Basis of Food Pairing in Indian Cuisine", 2015, http://arxiv.org/ftp/arxiv/papers/1502/1502.03815.pdf.

42 Concerns that sugar-laden fortified foods mask micronutrient dilution are reasonable, although the jury is out, and the American cranberry lobby is terrified by rules that might limit the use of sugar with their hyper-tart fruit. At any rate things can go in reverse as occurred with the ban on chocolate milk in some public schools, which led to sharp drops in the consumption of any milk at all and a corresponding increase in other beverages. This author has been through the Nesquik battle with his daughter, who fortunately still drinks milk and doesn't like any liquids with bubbles in them. For the analysis of who buys supplements, see Shaikh, Ulfat, *et al.*, "Vitamin and Mineral Supplement Use by Children and Adolescents in the 1999-2004 NHANES Survey", *Archives of Pediatrics and Adolescent Medicine*, 2009, Vol: 163:2, pp.150-157, http://www.ncbi.nlm.nih.gov/pmc/articles/PMC2996491/, DOI: 10.1001/archpediatrics.2008.523. For the analysis of fortified foods today, see Berner, Louise A., "Fortified Foods Are Major Contributors to Nutrient Intakes in Diets of US Children and Adolescents", *Journal of the Academy of Nutrition and Dietetics*, 2014, Vol. 114:7, pp. 1009-1022, http://www.andjrnl.org/article/S2212-2672(13)01609-2/fulltext, DOI: http://dx.doi.org/10.1016/j.jand.2013.10.012.

43 Cf. Rtveladze, Ketevan, *et al.*, "Health and Economic Burden of Obesity in Brazil", *Plos*, 2013, http://journals.plos.org/plosone/article?id=10.1371/journal.pone.0068785, DOI: 10.1371/journal.pone.0068785.

44 Cf. Pereira, Rosangela A., "Sources of Excessive Saturated Fat, Trans Fat and Sugar Consumption in Brazil: An Analysis of the First Brazilian Nationwide Individual Dietary Survey", *Public Health and Nutrition*, 2014, Vol. 17:1, pp. 113-121, DOI: 10.1017/S1368980012004892.

45 Sadam Satyanarayana and colleagues make the important point that food-processing is a dynamic process and not just one for established brands, which is likely more true for less-developed countries. See their "Potential Impacts of Food and its Processing on Global Sustainable Health", *Journal of Food Processing and Technology*, 2012, Vol. 3:2, http://www.omicsonline.org/potential-impacts-of-food-and-its-processing-on-global-sustainable-health-2157-7110.1000143.pdf, DOI: 10.4172/2157-7110.1000143. Beriberi, a pan-Asian calamity, turned out not to have an infectious vector but was caused by thiamine deficiency due to new industrial techniques of milling and polishing white rice. The problem was a lack, not a toxin. For a fine look at how colonial authorities struggled

with it at a time of paradigm changes in biology, see Arnold, David, "British India and the 'Beriberi Problem' 1798-1942", *Medical History*, 2010, Vol. 54:3, http://www.ncbi.nlm.nih.gov/pmc/articles/PMC2889456/.

46 "Bitter-sensitive children, however, ate 80% more broccoli with dressing than when served plain", and the richer the dressing, the more they ate. Cf. Fisher, J.O., "Offering 'Dip' Promotes Intake of a Moderately-liked Raw Vegetable Among Preschoolers with Genetic Sensitivity to Bitterness", *Journal of the Academy of Nutrition and Dietics*, 2012, Vol. 112:2, pp. 235-245, http://www.ncbi.nlm.nih.gov/pubmed/22741167.

47 Those observations have already produced medical advances of a sort, as it shows that some drugs that do not seem to pass human trials may in fact do so for heavy people, according to one research team working on ischemic stroke therapies. Cf. Yoon, Jeong Song, *et al.*, "Energy Restriction Negates NMDA Receptor Antagonist Efficacy in Ischemic Stroke", *NeuroMolecular Medicine*, Vol. 13:3, pp. 175-178, http://link.springer.com/article/10.1007%2Fs12017-011-8145-y. For Martin's report on rats, see Martin, Bronwen, *et al.*, "'Control' Laboratory Rodents are Metabolically Morbid: Why it Matters", *PNAS*, 2010, Vol. 107:14, pp. 6127-6133, http://www.pnas.org/content/107/14/6127.full, DOI: 10.1073/pnas.0912955107. For the Finnish paper on rye bread, see Lappi, Jenni, "Intake of Whole-Grain and Fiber-Rich Rye Bread Versus Refined Wheat Bread Does Not Differentiate Intestinal Microbiota Composition in Finnish Adults with Metabolic Syndrome", *Journal of Nutrition*, 2013, Vol. 143:5, pp. 648-655, http://jn.nutrition.org/content/143/5/648.full, DOI: 10.3945/jn.112.172668.

48 Wild-type humans with a reasonable risk appetite and living in reasonably complex environments do face extinction risks. For example, a public health official in Colorado has recently crunched the numbers and discovered that the main cause of concussions for youth playing soccer comes from heading the ball. Outlawing it has been suggested by a Boston-based nonprofit organization founded by a former professional wrestler. It turns out concussions are quite rare and two-thirds of them come from physical contact with another player. Cf. Comstock, Dawn, *et al.*, "An Evidence-Based Discussion of Heading the Ball and Concussions in High School Soccer", *JAMA Pediatrics*, 2015 http://archpedi.jamanetwork.com/article.aspx?articleid=2375128 DOI: 10.1001.jamapediatrics.2015/1062.

49 Cf. Vendruscolo, Leandro F., *et al.*, "Sugar Overconsumption during Adolescence Selectively Alters Motivation and Reward Function in Adult Rats", *Plos*, 2010, http://journals.plos.org/plosone/article?id=10.1371/journal.pone.0009296, DOI: 10.1371/journal.pone.0009296.

50 The upshot is that it is not just the medium – the screen – but the message that makes us overeat, according to Brian Wansink and his team at Cornell University. Cf., "Watch What You Eat: Action-Related Television Content Increases Food Intake", *JAMA Internal Medicine*, 2014, Vol. 174:11, pp. 1842-1843, http://archinte.jamanetwork.com/article.aspx?articleid=1899554, DOI: 10.1001/jamainternmed.2014.4098. For the theta burst study, see Lowe, Cassandra J. *et al.*, "The Effects of Theta Burst Stimulation to the Left Dorsolateral Prefrontal Cortex on Executive Function, Food Cravings and Snack Food Consumption", *Psychosomatic Medicine*, 2014, Vol. 76:7, pp. 503-511, http://journals.lww.com/psychosomaticmedicine/Abstract/2014/09000/The_Effects_of_Continuous_Theta_Burst_Stimulation.6.aspx, DOI: 10.1097/PSY.0000000000000090. For

the chronic stress study, see Tryon, M.S. *et al.*, "Chronic Stress Exposure May Affect the Brain's Response to High Calorie Food Cues and Predispose to Obesogenic Eating Habits", *Physiology and Behavior*, 2013, Vol. 120, pp. 233-242, http://www.ncbi.nlm.nih.gov/pubmed/23954410, DOI: 10.1016/j.physbeh.2013.08.010.

51 Martire, S.I. *et al.*, "Extended Exposure to A Palatable Cafeteria Diet Alters Gene Expression in Grain Regions Implicated in Reward, and Withdrawal from this Diet Alters Gene Expressions in Brain Regions Associated with Stress", *Behavioral Brain Research*, 2014, Vol. 265, pp. 132-141, http://www.sciencedirect.com/science/article/pii/S0166432814001028 DOI: 10.1016/j.bbr.2014.02.027. For the Beirut study, see Cf. Zeeni, N., *et al.*, "Environment Enrichment and Cafeteria Diet Attenuate the Response to Chronic Variable Stress in Rats", *Physiology and Behavior*, 2015, Vol. 139, pp. 41-49, http://www.ncbi.nlm.nih.gov/pubmed/25446213?dopt=Abstract, DOI: 10.1016/j.physbeh.2014.11.003.

Chapter 4

[1] While the biological dynamics outlined in Dr. Lustig's article of the same name has been taken down, this author appreciates the following premise: "Obesity is not the cause of metabolic syndrome; rather, it is a marker for the metabolic dysfunction that is occurring worldwide." Cf. "Fructose: It's 'Alcohol Without the Buzz", *Advances in Nutrition*, 2013, Vol. 4, pp. 226-235, http://advances.nutrition.org/content/4/2/226.full, DOI: 10.3945/an.112.002998.

[2] That there even is any correlation between HFCS and obesity is hardly clear, given that it is widely used in South Korea, where obesity is marginal, and barely used at all in Mexico, where obesity rates are the highest in the world. Cf. White, John S., "Misconceptions About High-Fructose Corn Syrup: Is It Uniquely Responsible for Obesity, Reactive Dicarbonyl Compounds, and Advanced Glycation Endproducts?" *Journal of Nutrition*, 2009, Vol. 139:6, pp. 1219-1227, http://jn.nutrition.org/content/139/6/1219S.full, DOI: 10.3945/jn.108.097998.

[3] One in four of those estimated deaths occurred in high-income countries. Cf. Singh, Gitanjali M., *et al.*, "Estimated Global, Regional, and National Disease Burdens Related to Sugar-Sweetened Beverage Consumption in 2010", *Circulation*, 2015, http://circ.ahajournals.org/content/early/2015/06/25/CIRCULATIONAHA.114.010636.abstract?-papetoc, DOI: 10.1161/circulationaha.114.010636 A common stylistic ploy of the sugar industry is to emphasize that there is no proof that their product is the "unique" cause of obesity. The American Beverage Association's response can be found here: http://www.prnewswire.com/news-releases/beverage-industry-responds-to-study-that-purports-to-link-beverages-to-global-disease-300106984.html.

[4] A chemical study of 23 popular soft drinks found that the HFCS used in some appeared to be as high as 65 percent fructose – which would make it sweeter – and that total sugar content varied from 85 to 128 percent of what was indicated on product labels. The overshoot was typically from fountain-served drinks at fast-food franchises, suggesting that the labels presume ice will be added. For the record, this study found that Pepsi had the highest fructose ratio, while the highest total sugars were found in "fruit juice" drinks such as Kern's Nectar Strawberry and Tampico Citrus Punch. The authors also report that they did not in fact find sucrose in Mexican Coca-Cola, which is popularly assumed to use cane sugar instead of HFCS. Cf. Ventura, Emily E., *et al.*, "Sugar Content of Popular Sweetened Beverages Based on Objective Laboratory Analysis: Focus on Fructose Content", *Obesity*, 2010, Vol. 19:4, pp. 868-874, http://onlinelibrary.wiley.com/doi/10.1038/oby.2010.255/abstract, DOI:10.1038/oby.2010.255. A later study found broadly similar results and also noted a much higher fructose level in a popular apple juice concoction. Apples are naturally rich in fructose. Cf. Walker, Ryan W., *et al.*, "Fructose Content in Popular Beverages Made With and Without High-fructose Corn Syrup", *Nutrition*, 2014, Vol. 30:7-8, pp. 928-935, http://www.sciencedirect.com/science/article/pii/S0899900714001920, DOI: 10.1016/j.nut.2014.04.003.

[5] Apart from that claim, an hour of television viewing translates to a 12 percent higher chance of obesity and only running an entire marathon would burn off the calories consumed from a double cheese burger with french fries, a soft drink and a dessert. Cf. "Ebbeling, Cara B., *et al.*, "Childhood Obesity: Public-health Crisis, Common

Sense Cure", *The Lancet*, 2002, Vol. 360, pp. 473-482, http://www.ncbi.nlm.nih.gov/pubmed/12241736.

6 One of the interesting findings of the study may be that people forced to consume so much fructose apparently cut back on carbohydrates but seek out extra fats. See Perez-Pozo, S.E., *et al.*, "Excessive Fructose Intake Induces the Features of Metabolic Syndrome in Healthy Adult Men: Role of Uric Acid in the Hypertensive Response", *International Journal of Obesity*, 2009, Vol. 34, pp. 454-461, http://www.nature.com/ijo/journal/v34/n3/full/ijo2009259a.html, DOI: 10.1038/ijo.2009.259.

7 Cf. Soenen, Stijn, *et al.*, "No Differences in Satiety or Energy Intake After High-fructose Corn Syrup, Sucrose or Milk Preloads", *American Journal of Clinical Nutrition*, 2007, Vol. 86:6, pp. 1586-1594, http://ajcn.nutrition.org/content/86/6/1586.long. The second study was done by the science advisor of an HFCS producer. Cf. Anderson, G. Harvey, "Much Ado About High-Fructose Corn Syrup in Beverages; The Meat of the Matter", *American Journal of Clinical Nutrition*, 2007, Vol.86:6, pp. 1577-1578, http://ajcn.nutrition.org/content/86/6/177.full.

8 HFCS's name came about because it was high in fructose in relation to regular corn syrup, not sugar. The industry's current legal effort to use the word sugar highlights how that might have been a commercially short-sighted decision, although it may have been chosen to distinguish itself from the word sugar, which cyclically falls out of favor. *The Times* noted that some critics say HFCS should not be considered natural because its molecular structure is not found in corn, being instead a syrup produced by enzymes that is then mixed with regular all-glucose corn syrup. Cf. Warner, Melanie, "A Sweetener With a Bad Rap", *The New York Times*, July 2, 2006.

9 The USDA has in fact been shifting some of its subsidizing power to the world of fresh produce, although the scale is miniscule compared to the well-entrenched cash flowing to the corn sector. As noted earlier in this book, it is removal of subsidies to sugar, not corn, that likely pose the greatest threat to HFCS's commercial viability. Cf. Duffey, Kiyah J. and Popkin, Barry M., "High-fructose Corn Syrup: Is this what's for Dinner?" *American Journal of Clinical Nutrition*, 2008, Vol. 88:6, pp. 1722-1732, http://ajcn.nutrition.org/content/88/6/1722S.full, DOI: 10.3945/ajcn.2008.25825C.

10 Having reviewed massive amounts of data and experiments, Tappy says there is "at present not a single hint that HFCS may have more deleterious effect on body weight than other sources of sugar." But he does see a legitimate need for more research on a possible role in metabolic diseases, particularly because it's not clear whether pure fructose acts differently than fructose bound to sugar, as it is in HFCS. In one of his experiments, pure fructose consumption elicited no real change in plasma glucose and insulin, but there was a sharp increase in net carbohydrate oxidation, part of which is likely to take place in the liver. Cf. Tappy, Luc and Lê Kim-Anne, "Metabolic Effects of Fructose and the Worldwide Increase in Obesity", *Physiological Reviews*, 2010, Vol. 90:1, pp. 230-246, http://physrev.physiology.org/content/90/1/23.long, DOI:10.1152/physrev.00019.2009.

11 Hitting the wall can cause lasting muscle fiber damage, so it's not just a psychological issue. The right technique for refuelling during high-performance sports events is a holy grail and the market is crowded with consultants and a slew of commercial products that are also available for spectators. One reason consensus is elusive is that everybody is different, or at least the amount of glycogen they can store in their leg muscles

is. Cf. Rapoport, Benjamin I., "Metabolic Factors Limiting Performance in Marathon Runners", *Plos*, 2010, http://journals.plos.org/ploscompbiol/article?id=10.1371/journal.pcbi.1000960, DOI:10.1371/journal.pcbi.1000960.

12 It's interesting that the Bantu, who had a low-fat, high-carbohydrate level, reacted so smoothly to a higher fat, high sugar diet. Cholesterol levels declined in all cases except for a few subjects who ate a lot of nuts, and so did triglyceride levels except for a brief period triggered by a shortage of avocados. The authors also note that the subjects had ad libitum access to as much sugar as they wanted, but expressed desire for salt. Cf. Meyer, B.J., *et al.*, "Some Biochemical Effects of a Mainly Fruit diet in Man", *South African Medical Journal*, 1971, Vol. 45:10, pp. 253-61, http://www.ncbi.nlm.nih.gov/pubmed/5573330.

13 Sumathi Reddy reported on some such gadgets, including a $99 Chinese fork that vibrates if your bites are more than 10 seconds apart and a $250 "talking" plate that measures how fast you eat and tells you how full you should feel. She also mentioned an app being developed at a US university designed to help people chew 100 times a day. That's based on the notion that men take in 17 calories per bite on average and women 11. In case anyone cares, that would be well below the basal metabolism rate even for a five-foot, 100-pound 20-year-old girl. Reddy also noted a Chinese study establishing that chewing 40 times before swallowing cuts calorie intake by 12 percent compared to doing so only 15 times. See her article "How May Bites Do You Take a Day? Try for 100", *Wall Street Journal*, Aug. 11, 2014, http://www.wsj.com/articles/how-many-bites-do-you-take-a-day-try-for-100-1407798123.

14 The python experiment was done by biologists and anthropologists at Harvard University who think that the energy efficiencies of cooked food marked a key moment in human evolution as it represented a technology that externalized part of the digestive process. They calculate that cooking increases the energy harvested from potatoes by more than 30 percent, and by almost 15 percent for wheat. Gains from cooking are larger than those from beating fibrous foods as we once did and primates still do. Interestingly, they also found that cooking an egg increases the digestibility of its protein content by 45 percent to 78 percent. Cf. Carmody, Rachel N. and Wrangham, Richard W., "The energetic significance of cooking", *Journal of Human Evolution*, 2009, Vol. 57:4, pp. 379-391, http://www.ncbi.nlm.nih.gov/pubmed/19732938, DOI: 10.1016/j.jhevol.2009.02.011.

15 The evening chats engage "big picture" ideas, implying that culture and language may have been born not from the need to transmit technical instructions directly from imagination, says Polly Wiessner. See her "Embers of Society: Firefight Among the Ju/'hoansi Bushmen", *PNAS*, 2014, Vol. 111:39, pp. 14027-14035, http://www.pnas.org/content/111/39/14027.full, DOI: 10.1073/pnas.1404212111.

16 Not much is known about the US Flavor and Extract Manufacturers Association, the relevant industry lobby with a $5 million operating budget and members ranging from well-known brands to Gingko Bioworks, which operates the world's largest "organism foundry" in Boston, and Givaudan, a Swiss firm that sells around $5 billion in flavors and aromas a year, many aiming to offer the "comfort of indulgence" to sweet products. The group has declared more than 2,700 flavoring chemicals safe in the past five decades. These are routinely reviewed by international bodies. See "Food Flavor System a 'Black Box'", The Center for Public Integrity, June 9, 2015, http://www.publicintegrity.org/2015/06/09/17465/food-flavor-safety-system-black-box.

[17] Underscoring how little is known, some Maillard reactions, such as with coffee, appear to have positive antioxidant effects. Cf. Tuohy, Kieran M., "Metabolism of Maillard Reaction Products by the Human Gut Microbiota-implications for Health", *Molecular Nutrition and Food Research Journal*, 2007, Vol. 50, pp. 847-857, http://www.ncbi.nlm.nih.gov/pubmed/16671057, DOI:10.1002/mnfr.200500126.

[18] The scientists note that there may even be "early glycation endproducts", and also that some may even have beneficial effects. Cf. Poulsen, Malene W., *et al.*, "Advanced Glycation Endproducts in Food and their Effects on Health", *Food and Chemical Toxicology*, 203, Vol. 60, pp. 10-37, http://www.ncbi.nlm.nih.gov/pubmed/23867544 DOI: 10.1016/j.fct.2013.06.052.

[19] The list goes on and includes 549 foods. On a per serving basis, AGEs are particularly present in nuts of all kinds, with pine nuts in the lead, sesame oil, Italian Pinot Grigio wine, dried figs, Big Macs and pizza, broiled as opposed to boiled hot dogs, cold-cut meats, oven-fried chicken breast (even more than a serving of "McNuggets"), bacon, higher-trophic fish such as tuna and salmon, sautéed tofu, and croissants. Curiously, a breakfast cereal billed as high in fiber had six times as much as standard corn flakes, and "Cheez Doodles" had six times more than Doritos corn chips, which may reflect the manufacturers' insistence on short shelf lives for the latter product. Those who wish to avoid AGEs should consider stewing their meat and eating more fresh produce, the researchers note. Cf. Uribarri, Jaime, *et al.*, "Advanced Glycation End Products in Foods and a Practical Guide to their Reduction in the Diet", *Journal of the American Dietetic Association*, 2010, Vol. 110:6, http://www.ncbi.nlm.nih.gov/pmc/articles/PMC3704564/, DOI: 10.1016/j.jada.2010.03.018.

[20] Cai, Weijing, *et al.*, "Oral Advanced Glycation Endproducts (AGEs) Promote Insulin Resistance and Diabetes by Depleting the Antioxidant Defenses AGE Receptor-1 and Sirtuin 1", *PNAS*, 2012, http://www.ncbi.nlm.nih.gov/pmc/articles/PMC3465382/, DOI: 10.1073/pnas.1205847109.

[21] Also of interest is that fructose is not involved in this kind of glycation. One of the authors of this study was the author of the impressive review of AGEs and a person who had hoped to find evidence incriminating fructose. Cf. Budek Mark, Alicja, *et al.*, "Consumption of a Diet Low in Advanced Glycation End Products for 4 Weeks Improves Insulin Sensitivity in Overweight Women", *Diabetes Care*, 2014, Vol. 37:1, pp. 88-95, http://care.diabetesjournals.org/content/37/1/88.long, DOI: 10.2337/dc13-0842. Also see Forbes, Josephine M., *et al.*, "Below the Radar: Advanced Glycation End Products that Detour 'around the side'", *Clinical Biochemistry Review*, 2005, Vol. 26:4, pp. 123-134, http://www.ncbi.nlm.nih.gov/pmc/articles/PMC1320176/.

Chapter 5

1 From "Foods: Nutritive Value and Cost", *Farmers Bulletin*, No. 23, US Department of Agriculture, 1894, http://www.ars.usda.gov/SP2UserFiles/Place/80400530/pdf/hist/oes_1894_farm_bul_23.pdf.

2 The original calculation was made by Thomas D. Luckey of the University of Missouri at a conference he organized in a bid to galvanize interest in intestinal microecology. That fact was uncovered by NIH researcher Judah Rosner who argued that credible estimates of just how many microorganisms we house and how many cells make up the human body vary enormously – the first by a factor of 13 and the second by a factor of 36 – so that instead of 10 the number could be 80, or even only 0.04. An informal consensus appears to be settling on a ratio of three, according to the wry reporting of Peter Andrey Smith, who tells that Luckey was a doll-collecting rattlesnake-milker who believed low doses of radiation were good for you and lived until 94. As it happens, he was also the first scientist to show that livestock given non-therapeutic antibiotics would put on weight faster, a discovery that has led to an estimated 3 million kilograms of antibiotics, or 80 percent of all such drugs used in the USA, being fed to promote fatter cows, poultry, and pigs. That's not, however, why chickens today are four times bigger than they were in the 1950s, according to a study funded by the poultry industry. That research found that the typical 4.2 kilogram broiler chicken is bigger than its 905 gram ancestor in 1957 due to farmers' selecting for genetic traits. Today's chickens also eat only half as much per unit of flesh as their forebears. Cf. Smith, "Is Your Body Mostly Microbes? Actually, We Have No Idea", *The Boston Globe*, Sept. 14, 2014, https://www.bostonglobe.com/ideas/2014/09/13/your-body-mostly-microbes-actually-have-idea/qlcoKot4wfUXecjeVaFKFN/story.html, and Zuidhof, Martin, *et al.*, "Growth, Efficiency and Yield of Commercial Broilers from 1957, 1978 and 2005", *Poultry Science*, 2014, Vol. 93, pp. 2970-2982, http://ps.oxfordjournals.org/content/93/12/2970.full.pdf+html?sid=c660528f-969d-418d-92d5-0102d6861a82.

3 The researchers, Eric A. Franzosa and colleagues, suggest this may one day pose thorny questions about privacy. See their "Identifying Personal Microbiomes Using Metagenomics Codes", *PNAS*, 2015, Vol. 112:22, http://www.pnas.org/content/112/22/E2930.abstract, DOI: 10.1073/pnas.1423854112.

4 Cancer treatments such as chemotherapy and radiation often annihilate gut biota, which is now seen as a major reason patients are often weak and lack immunity. Doctors are now increasingly prescribing fecal self-transplants so that patients can restore their live-in community after treatment.

5 The doctors, Neha Alang and Colleen R. Kelly, have decided to adopt a policy to use non-obese donors for fecal transplants in the future. See their "Weight Gain After Fecal Microbiota Transplantation", *Open Forum Infectious Diseases*, 2015, Vol. 2:1, http://ofid.oxfordjournals.org/content/2/1/ofv004.full, DOI: 10.1093/ofid/ofv004.

6 The researchers conducted an intense survey of other inhabitants of the mouse guts, finding one group that had never been detected before and which they suggested may be descendants of non-photosynthetic cyanobacteria that, while now adapted to life inside animals, were essentially creatures of the dark that "could shed light on the great oxygenation event that occurred 2.2 billion years ago, when Cyanobacteria

profoundly changed the chemistry of the Earth's atmosphere." Cyanobacteria are the world's oldest known fossils and their progeny are busy nitrogen fixers all over the planet as well as giving pink flamingos their color. They are believed to have served as godparents to biodiversity in a long-ago deal with plants where they offered to make food for eukaryote cells in exchange for housing – a deal they have evidently extended to the animal kingdom. Cf. Ley, R.E., *et al.* "Obesity Alters Gut Microbial Ecology", *PNAS*, 2005, Vol. 102:3, pp. 11070-11075, http://www.ncbi.nlm.nih.gov/pubmed//16033867, DOI: 10.1073/pnas.0504978102.

7 Cf. Jumpertz, Reiner, *et al.*, "Energy-balance Studies Reveal Associations Between Gut Microbes, Caloric Load, and Nutrient Absorption in Humans", *American Journal of Clinical Nutrition*, 2011, Vol. 94:1, pp. 58-65, http://www.ncbi.nlm.nih.gov/pmc/articles/PMC3127503/, DOI: 10.3945/ajcn.110.010132.

8 Backhed, Fredrik, "Mechanisms Underlying the Resistance to Diet-induced Obesity in Germ-free Mice", *PNAS*, 2006, Vol. 104:3, pp. 979-984, http://www.pnas.org/content/104/3/979.full, DOI: 10.0173/pnas/060374104.

9 Cf. Scott, Karen A., *et al.*, "Manipulating the Gut Microbiota to Maintain Health and Treat Disease", *Microbial Ecology*, 2015, Vol. 26, http://www.ncbi.nlm.nih.gov/pmc/articles/PMC4315778/, DOI: 10.3402/mehd.v26.25877.

10 Csergo, Julia, "Food Consumption and Risk of Obesity: The Medical Discourse in France 1850-1930", in Oddy, Derek J., ed., *The Rise of Obesity in Europe*, Ashgate, 2009.

11 Ellekilde, *et al.*, "Transfer of Gut Microbiota from Lean and Obese Mice to Antibiotic-treated Mice", *Scientific Reports*, 2014, Vol. 4, http://www.nature.com/srep/2014/140801/srep05922/full/srep05922.html, DOI: 10.1038/srep05922.

12 Ridaura, Vanessa K., et al, "Cultured Gut Microbiota from Twins Discordant for Obesity Modulate Adiposity and Metabolic Phenotypes in Mice", *Science*, 2013, Vol. 341, p. 6150, http://www.ncbi.nlm.nih.gov/pmc/articles/PMC3829625/, DOI: 10.1126/science.1241214.

13 Cf. Turnbaugh, Peter J. and Gordon, Jeffrey I., "The Core Gut Microbiome, Energy Balance and Obesity", *Journal of Physiology*, 2009, vol. 598, pp. 4153-4158, http://www.ncbi.nlm.nih.gov/pmc/articles/PMC2754355/, DOI: 10.1113/jphysiol.2009.174136, and Turnbaugh, Peter J. *et al.*, "The Effect of Diet on the Human Microbiome; A Metagenomic Analysis in Humanized Gnotobiotic Mice", *Science Translational Medicine*, 2009, Vol. 11 http://www.ncbi.nlm.nih.gov/pmc/articles/PMC2894525/ DOI: 10.1126/scitranslmed.3000322.

14 Cf. Vreize, A., *et al.*, "Transfer of Intestinal Microbiota from Lean Donors Increases Insulin Sensitivity in Individuals with Metabolic Syndrome", *Gastroenterology*, 2012, Vol. 143:4, pp. 913-916, http://www.ncbi.nlm.nih.gov/pubmed/22728514 DOI: 10.1053/j.gastro.2012.06.031.

15 Antibiotic therapy itself, common in western and many other countries, can obviously alter the microbiota and in fact increase diabetes risk. A review of more than 208,000 diabetic cases, and almost a million people in total, found that treatment not with just one but with two to five antibiotic courses in a single year was associated with increased risk of diabetes. Cf. Boursi, Ben, *et al.*, "The Effect of Past Antibiotic Exposure on Diabetes Risk", *European Journal of Endocrinology*, 2015, Vol. 172, pp. 639-648, http://www.eje-online.org/content/172/6/639.abstract, DOI: 10.1530/EJE-14-1163.

[16] Cf. Hansen, Camilla H.F., *et al.*, "Mode of Delivery Shapes Gut Colonization Pattern and Modulates Regulatory Immunity in Mice", *The Journal of Immunology*, 2014, http://www.jimmunol.org/content/early/2014/06/19/jimmunol.1400085.full.pdf+html, DOI: 10.4049/jimmunol.1400085.

[17] Cf. Mueller, N.T., *et al.*, "Prenatal Exposure to Antibiotics, Cesarean Section and Risk of Childhood Obesity", *International Journal of Obesity*, 2014, Vol. 39:4, http://www.nature.com/ijo/journal/v39/n4/full/ijo2014180a.html, DOI: 10.1038/ijo.2014.180.

[18] Keep calm! A 20 percent greater chance translates, in the USA, to a 19.4 percent chance a C-section baby becomes obese as a child, compared to a 15.8 percent chance for a vaginally delivered baby. Cf. Cardwell, C.R., "Caesarean Section is Associated with an Increased Risk of Childhood-onset Type 1 Diabetes Mellitus: A Meta-Analysis of Observational Studies", *Diabetologia*, 2008, Vol. 51:5, pp. 726-35, http://www.ncbi.nlm.nih.gov/pubmed/18292986, DOI 10.1007/s00125-008-0941-z.

[19] In their thorough review, Josef Neu and Jona Rushing note that the bacteria works with the gut mucosa to produce antibodies to pathogens while tolerating – a learned behavior especially in the first year of a person's life – the helpful microbial species as "old friends." They note bacteria can also influence oral tolerance, which instructs the immune system to be less sensitive to certain antigens once ingested, including those produced by gut bacteria, thereby pre-emptively lowering the frequency and intensity of aggressive immune responses such as those that trigger allergies and autoimmune disease. They also cite a study that found a host of pathogens in hospitals often pry their way into a C-section baby's microbiome. Cf. their "Caesarean versus Vaginal Delivery: Long-term Infant Outcomes and the Hygiene Hypothesis", *Clinical Perinatology*, 2011, Vol. 38:2, pp. 321-331, http://www.ncbi.nlm.nih.gov/pmc/articles/PMC3110651/, DOI: 10.1016/j.clp.2011.03.008.

[20] Blaser also notes that infant formulas "may not have been constructed with the benefit of millions of years of mammalian evolution, because breast milk contains nutrients that specifically select for the growth of preferred coevolved organisms and inhibits opportunists and pathogens." See his "Like Genes, Our Microbes Pass from Parent to Child", *Scientific American*, Feb. 17, 2015, http://www.scientificamerican.com/article/like-genes-our-microbes-pass-from-parent-to-child/.

[21] In a global report, the WHO found there are 6 million C-sections too many and at the same time 3 million too few, reflecting a calculation based on excessive use of the practice in wealthier countries and the low rates in some poorer nations. Cf. Gibbons, Luz, *et al.*, "The Global Numbers and Costs of Additionally Needed and Unnecessary Caesarean Sections Performed per Year: Overuse as a Barrier to Universal Coverage", WHO, 2010, http://www.who.int/healthsystems/topics/financing/healthreport/30C-sectioncosts.pdf. Also see Lauer, Jeremy A., *et al.*, "Determinants of Caesarean Section Rates in Developed Countries: Supply, Demand and Opportunities for Control", WHO, 2010, http://www.who.int/healthsystems/topics/financing/healthreport/29DeterminantsC-section.pdf.

[22] One American woman recently wrote a column on her surprise at the pressure she was put under to have a C-section. And when eventually she didn't, she felt as if the hospital ward was unprepared for a natural delivery. Interestingly, the woman herself is an expert in the field of medical education, underscoring the potential gap between policy theo-

reticians and actual practice. Cf. Keirns, Carla C., "I didn't realize the pressure to have a C-section until I was about to deliver", *Washington Post*, Jan. 5, 2015, http://www.washingtonpost.com/national/health-science/pregnant-doctor-finds-intense-pressure-to-have-a-caesarean-delivery/2015/01/05/949ed918-7bd3-11e4-84d4-7c896b90abdc_story.html.

[23] A new Danish study found a strong correlation between C-section births and later chronic diseases on the basis of a survey of 2 million people born from 1973 to 2012, making it one of the largest epidemiological correlation studies ever. Cf. Ringgaard, Anne, "Giant Study Links C-sections with Chronic Disorders", Dec. 9, 2014, http://sciencenordic.com/giant-study-links-c-sections-chronic-disorders.

[24] Indication of a C-section on birth certificates was introduced in 2003, and 41 states had implemented the rule a decade later. The US C-section rate varies enormously, with a low of 22 percent in Utah and 38 percent in New Jersey in 2007. The practice has been subsiding in recent years after a very rapid increase in the decade from the mid-1990s. See Barber, Emma L. et al, "Contributing Indications to the Rising Cesarean Delivery Rate", *Obstetrics & Gynecology*, 2013, Vol. 118:1, pp. 29-38, http://www.ncbi.nlm.nih.gov/pmc/articles/PMC3751192/, DOI: 10.1097/AOG.Ob013e31821e5f65.

[25] The authors note that doctors reported a modest concern about litigation but none about economic incentives. They also warn that C-section requests may be driven by "media-publicized fashionable trends featuring vaginal delivery as unsafe, archaic, disfiguring and ultimately socially unacceptable." Given that C-sections are increasing fastest for women at the lowest risk, such factors would appear relevant. They also note that cultural factors can include relative enthusiasm for technology, noting that 46 percent of US obstetricians would favor a C-section for themselves. Cf. Habiba, M., *et al.*, "Caesarean Section on Request: A Comparison of Obstetricians' Attitudes in Eight European Countries", *BJOG*, 2006, http://onlinelibrary.wiley.com/doi/10.1111/j.1471-0528.2006.00933.x/full, DOI: 10.1111/j.1471-0528.2006.00933.x.

[26] The remarkable increase in C-sections at the hospital in Dar es Salaam did not reflect any increase in mothers who had already undergone the operation, nor were low-weight babies more frequent than usual in the area. Maternal mortality rates actually rose. Cf. Litorp, Helena, *et al.*, "Increasing Caesarean Selection Rates Among Low-Risk Groups: A Panel Study Classifying Deliveries According to Robston at a University Hospital in Tanzania", *BMC Pregnancy and Childbirth*, 2013, Vol. 13, http://www.biomedcentral.com/1471-2393/13/107, DOI: 10.1186/1471-2393-13-107.

[27] Cf. Texeira, Cristina, *et al.*, "The Brazilian Preference: Cesarean Delivery among Immigrants in Portugal", *Plos*, 2013, http://journals.plos.org/plosone/article?id=10.1371/journal.pone.0060168, DOI: 0.1371/journal.pone.0060168.

[28] Women in all the countries tended to think highly of themselves compared to foreigners, but the outliers were Brazil on the high end and Japan on the low end. Cf. Etcoff, Nancy, *et al.*, "The Real Truth About Beauty", commissioned by Dove, a Unilever beauty brand, 2004, http://www.clubofamsterdam.com/contentarticles/52%20Beauty/dove_white_paper_final.pdf.

[29] Zlot, Al, *et al.*, "Association of Acculturation with Cesarean Section among Latinas", *Maternal Child Health Journal*, 2005, Vol. 9:1, pp. 11-20, http://www.ncbi.nlm.nih.gov/pubmed/15880970.

[30] The study raised "changes in the gut microbiome" to one of the four most likely explanatory candidates, placing it alongside mainstays such as increased calorie intake, changes in the composition of diet, and sedentary lifestyles. Cf. Ng, Marie, *et al.*, "Global, Regional, and National Prevalence of Overweight and Obesity in Children and Adults During 1980-2013: A Systematic Analysis for the Global Burden of Disease Study 2013", *The Lancet*, Vol. 384:9945, pp. 766-781, http://www.thelancet.com/journals/lancet/article/PIIS0140-6736(14)60460-8/fulltext, DOI: http://dx.doi.org/10.1016/S0140-6736(14)60460-8.

[31] The bacteria using choline from protein for energy were involved in the production of trimethylamine N-oxide, or TMAO, which has been shown to exacerbate impaired glucose tolerance and obstructs the way insulin signals are sent and received, at least in mice fed high-fat diets.

[32] Zhao's team said its typical diet in the experiment included appropriate amounts of vegetables, fruits, and nuts and three formulas made by a Chinese maker of pre-prepared foods called Perfect. Of these, Formula No. 1, designed to help satisfy hunger pains, was a gruel made of 12 component materials from whole grains and fiber-rich plants known in traditional Chinese medicine including oats, buckwheat, yellow corn, red and white beans, yams, peanuts, lotus seed, and wolfberry. Each can had 69 grams of carbohydrates, 15 grams of protein, 5 grams of fat and 6 grams of fiber and packed 336 kilocalories. Formula No. 2, given once a day, was an infusion powder containing bitter melon and oligosaccharides. No. 3, given at least once a day, was an infusion powder containing soluble prebiotics. The dietary treatment cut total calorie intake by 30 percent but raised the share provided by carbohydrates. Whole grains also displaced white rice as the primary carbohydrate source.

[33] Cf. Englyst, K.N., *et al.*, "Nutritional Characterization and Measurement of Dietary Carbohydrates", *European Journal of Clinical Nutrition*, 2007, Vol. 61, pp. 19-39, http://www.nature.com/ejcn/journal/v61/n1s/full/1602937a.html, DOI:10.1038/sj.ejcn.1602937.

[34] Beyond being overwhelmingly sucrose, honey contains minerals such as zinc, potassium, and manganese as well as phenolic compounds, flavonoids, organic acids, carotenoid-derived compounds, ascorbic acid, vitamins, and more items modern industry also synthesizes. Gut studies show that honey augments the growth of Bifidobacterium species, while it also improves fat metabolism, has led to weight loss in people and sheep and, surprisingly given its sugar content, has proven hypoglycemic in diabetic rats. Cf., Omotayo, O., *et al.*, "Honey – A Novel Antidiabetic Agent", *International Journal of Biological Sciences*, 2012, Vol. 8:6, pp. 913-934, http://www.ncbi.nlm.nih.gov/pmc/articles/PMC3399220/, DOI:10.7150/ijbs.3697, and "Effect of Honey in Diabetes Mellitus: Matters Arising", *Journal of Diabetes & Metabolic Disorders*, 2014, Vol. 13, http://www.ncbi.nlm.nih.gov/pmc/articles/PMC3909917/, DOI: 10.1186/2251-6581-13-23.

[35] Cf. Suez, Jotham, *et al.*, "Artificial Sweeteners Induce Glucose Intolerance by Altering the Gut Microbiota", *Nature*, 2014, Vol. 514, pp. 181-186, http://www.nature.com/nature/journal/v514/n7521/full/nature13793.html, DOI:10.1038/nature13793.

[36] Cf. Chassaing, Benoit, *et al.*, "Dietary Emulsifiers Impact the Mouse Gut Microbiota Promoting Colitis and Metabolic Syndrome", *Nature*, 2015, Vol. 519, pp. 92-96, http://www.nature.com/nature/journal/v519/n7541/full/nature14232.html, DOI:10.1038/nature14232.

[37] Cf. Jaeggi, T., *et al.*, "Iron Fortification Adversely Affects the Gut Microbiome, Increases Pathogenic Abundance and Induces Intestinal Kenyan Infants", *Gut*, 2015, Vol. 64:5, pp. 731-42, http://www.ncbi.nlm.nih.gov/pubmed/25143342, DOI: 10.1136/gutjnl-2014-307720.

[38] Cf. De Filippo, Carlotta De, *et al.*, "Impact of Diet Shaping Gut Microbiota Revealed by a Comparative Study in Children from Europe and Rural Africa", *PNAS*, 2010, Vol. 107:33, pp. 14691-14696, http://www.pnas.org/content/107/33/14691.full, DOI: 10.1073/pnas.1005963107.

[39] Cf. Cotillard, Aurélie and Kennedy, Sean, "Dietary Intervention Impact on Gut microbial Gene Richness", *Nature*, 2013, Vol. 500, pp. 585-588, http://www.nature.com/nature/journal/v500/n7464/full/nature12480.html, DOI: 10.1038/nature12480.

[40] Ironically, children who are born underweight appear to be programmed to catch up if possible, a process that requires a metabolic regulatory system that has a high tendency to lead to obesity later, raising the spectre of a dreadful paradox in which an economic boom might prove disastrous for people's longer-term health not just because of their transition to a richer diet but due to their having started with a poorer one.

[41] In their 1985 report, *Energy and Protein Requirements*, FAO and WHO said the basal metabolic rate for children of the age in the study is 22.7 times their weight plus 495 calories. Assuming a 5-year-old weighing 18 kilograms – typical for an industrialized economy – that would be about 900 calories. The study reports that Burkina Faso kids were consuming around 1,000 calories a day, while the ones in Florence were consuming 1,500 calories. Energy requirements for adults vary according to their activity, and measure around 1.5 times the basal metabolic rate for a wealthy housewife or retiree and well above 2 times for a working male.

[42] US consumption of food prepared away from home rose to 32 percent of calories in 2008, up from 18 percent in 1977, while in cash terms it rose to 43.1 percent in 2012 from 25.9 percent in 1970, according to the Department of Agriculture, which ventured that food prepared out of the home tends, in America, to be low in fiber and other nutrients the gut biota needs. For the Hazda, see Crittenden, Alyssa, *et al.*, "Gut Microbiome of the Hazda Hunter-gatherers", *Nature Communications*, 2014, Vol. 5, http://www.nature.com/ncomms/2014/140415/ncomms4654/full/ncomms4654.html, DOI 10.1038/ncomm4654.

[43] A detailed study of the three tubers most commonly eaten by the Hazda showed they consisted of up to 48 percent simple sugars, 26 percent starch and from 2 to 7 percent protein. Cf. Schoeninger, Margaret J., et al, "Composition of Tubers Used by Hazda Foragers of Tanzania", *Journal of Food Composition and Analysis*, 2001, Vol. 14:1, pp. 15-25, http://www.sciencedirect.com/science/article/pii/S088915750090961X.

[44] Precisely because the Hazda are so well-adjusted to their size and diet, they would not be able to burn the extra calories of the dreaded western diet if inundated with energy-dense, nutrient-poor, highly-processed foods. Australian Aboriginals forced to transition into the imposed sedentary life of a quasi-reservation setting lost both their native diet and microbiome and their energy balance, and now endure an appalling incidence of diabetes and obesity. Farming communities are the one sociological type that really do have higher total energy expenditure than others. That said, humans

by nature have low energy expenditure compared to other mammals, possibly linked to lower predation risk. Cf. Pontzer, Herman, *et al.*, "Hunter-gatherer Energetics and Human Obesity", *Plos*, 2012 http://journals.plos.org/plosone/article?id=10.1371/journal.pone.0040503, DOI: 10.1371/journal.pone.0040503.

[45] Cf. Ichikawa, Mitsuo, "Ecological and Sociological Importance of Honey to the Mbuti Net Hunter, Eastern Zaire", manuscript, http://jambo.africa.kyoto-u.ac.jp/kiroku/asm_normal/abstracts/pdf/ASM%20%20Vol.1%201981/Mitsuo%20ICHIKAWA.pdf.

[46] Cf. Eteraf-Oskouei, Tahereh, "Traditional and Modern Uses of Natural Honey in Human Diseases: A Review", *Iran Journal of Basic Medical Science*, 2013, Vol. 16:6, pp. 731-742, http://www.ncbi.nlm.nih.gov/pmc/articles/PMC3758027/.

[47] This laboratory in what is now Silicon Valley also treated cases of extreme obesity, putting them on a "total starvation diet" that led them to have only one "very small" bowel movement a month. Cf. Attebery, H.R., *et al.*, "Effect of a Chemically Defined Diet on Normal Human Fecal Flora", *The American Journal of Clinical Nutrition*, 1972, Vol. 25:12, pp. 1391-1398, http://ajcn.nutrition.org/content/25/12/1391.long.

[48] Cf. Clarke, Siobhan F., "Exercise and Associated Dietary Extremes Impact on Gut Microbial Diversity", *Gut*, 2014, Vol. 63, pp. 1913-1920, http://www.ncbi.nlm.nih.gov/pubmed/25021423, DOI: 10.1136/gutjnl-2013-30654.

[49] Here is the breakthrough study: Everard, Amandine, *et al.*, "Cross-talk Between Akkermansia Muciniphila and Intestinal Epithelium Controls Diet-induced Obesity", *PNAS*, 2013, Vol. 110:22, pp. 9066-9071, http://www.pnas.org/content/110/22/9066.full, DOI: 10.1073/pnas.1219451110. Liping Zhao also thinks *A. muciniphila* marks the point where microbiologists will move beyond the correlation so well known to epidemologists and into causality. See his landmark essay, "The Gut Microbiota and Obesity: From Correlation to Causality", *Nature Reviews Microbiology*, 2013, Vol. 11, pp. 639-647, http://www.nature.com/nrmicro/journal/v11/n9/abs/nrmicro3089.html, DOI: 10.1038/nrmicro3089. There have also, however, been reports that *A. muciniphila* can damage the gut wall in some situations, highlighting the need to calibrate its ideal abundance. Cf. Ganesh, Bhanu Priya, *et al.*, "Commensal Akkermansia muciniphila Exacerbates Gut Inflammation in Salmonella Typhimurium-Infected Gnotobiotic Mice", *Plos*, 2013, http://journals.plos.org/plosone/article?id=10.1371/journal.pones.0074963, DOI: 10.1371/journal.pone.0074963.

[50] Cf. Xue, Zhenghsheng, *et al.*, "The Bamboo-Eating Giant Panda Harbors a Carnivore-like Gut Microbiota, with Excessive Seasonal Variations", *mBio*, 2015, Vol. 6:3, http://mbio.asm.org/content/6/3/e00022-15.full, DOI: 10.1128/mBio.00022-1519, and Wei, Fuwen and Hu, Yibo, "Giant Pandas are not an Evolutionary Cul-de-sac", *Molecular Biology & Evolution*, 2015, Vol. 32:1, pp. 4-12, http://mbe.oxfordjournals.org/content/32/1/4.full, DOI: 10.1093/molbev/msu278, and Ley, Ruth E., *et al.*, "Evolution of Mammals and their Gut Microbes", *Science*, 2008, http://www.ncbi.nlm.nih.gov/pmc/articles/PMC2649005/, DOI 10.1126/science.1155725.

[51] *Polycarpa mytiligera*, an abundant tropical sea squirt known to accumulate heavy metals, has the opposite approach to the panda. It periodically punctures itself and tosses out most of its gut, which it then rebuilds. This is a defensive move that works because predatory fish find the eviscerated tissue repellent. Scientists hope that further study

of how the *Polycarpa* rebuilds its digestive tract in a matter of days will yield practical insights applicable to the human digestive tract. See Shenkar, Noa and Gordon, Tal, "Gut-spilling in Chordates: Evisceration in the Tropical Ascidian Polycarpa mytiligera", *Scientific Reports*, 2015, http://www.nature.com/srep/2015/150410/srep09614/full/srep09614.html, DOI:10.1038/srep09614.

Chapter 6

1 The quote continues, "Creating new names and assessments and apparent truths is enough to create new 'things'... Only a fool would think it was enough to point to this misty mantle of illusion in order to destroy the world that counts as essential." *The Gay Science*, tr. Walter Kaufmann, Random House.

2 Many of the Cree and Blackfeet people felt that they had less access to self-sufficiency than other communities in Canada's federalist system, sometimes saying they were "stuck in a corner" or even "sabotaged no matter what." A recurring theme was also that First Nations had lost many assets under colonialism and that forced attendance of residential schools had been a disaster for their cultures wherein children from the age of 4 were given a number and a uniform for 14 years, dug graves for their peers who died, suffered sexual abuse, and emerged with a host of psychological disorders – and that even recognition of this was routinely suppressed from the national discourse. Oster's research found that diabetes prevalence ranged from 1.2 to 18.3 percent among the 31 First Nations communities covered in the research, again underscoring how broad epidemiological surveys can miss critical points. To read the full paper, see Oster, Richard T., *et al.*, "Cultural Continuity, Traditional Indigenous Language, and Diabetes in Alberta First Nations: A Mixed Methods Study", *International Journal For Equity in Health*, 2014, Vol. 13, http://www.equityhealthj.com/content/13/1/92, DOI:10.1186/s12939-014-0092-4.

3 Residential students were chastised for scrounging for animal food in the barn as late as 1953, and one study presented in 1952 – which ended up inducing anemia in students over the following five years – was published with the usual rider that more such research was needed. See Mosby, Ian, "Administering Colonial Science: Nutrition Research and Human Biomedical Experimentation in Aboriginal Communities and Residential Schools, 1942-1952", *Histoire Sociale*, 2013, Vol. 46:91, pp. 144-172, http://www.fns.bc.ca/pdf/AdministeringSocialScience.mosby.pdf, DOI: 10.1353/his.2013.0015. Conducting life-threatening research on uninformed subjects was routine in the USA, and willingly published by academic journals, until Henry Beecher's article denouncing the practice in 1966, almost two decades after the Nuremberg trial of Nazi doctors accused of atrocities. See his "Ethics and Clinical Practice", *New England Journal of Medicine*, 1966, Vol. 274, http://www.hhs.gov/ohrp/archive/documents/BeecherArticle.pdf.

4 Oster noted that indigenous peoples themselves don't feel their logic is that of the victim. "Everybody has to feel like they're part of something. And if you don't, where are you going to end up? Probably on the street and homeless because you think nobody cares. And that's not just Aboriginal people, that's all people."

5 In separate work among Anishinaabe adults in Manitoba, Linda Garro had shown that the heath care message of individual responsibility for diabetes is short-sighted given the extent to which those suffering from it themselves regularly speak of environmental and social upheavals. See her "Individual or Societal Responsibility? Explanations of Diabetes in an Anishinaabe (Ojibwa) Community", *Social Science and Medicine*, Vol. 40:1, pp. 37-46, http://www.sciencedirect.com/science/article/pii/027795369400125D.

6 One of his salient points is that culture takes on increasing urgency as a conceptual tool whenever income inequality appears to be on its own less predictive of health

disparities. He concludes by warning that an economic emphasis on consumption constitutes "cultural fraud", essentially the system-wide promotion of ostensibly desirable lifestyles that are not in fact enjoyable. Cf. Eckersley, Richard, "Is Modern Western Culture a Health Hazard?" *International Journal of Epidemiology*, 2006, Vol. 35:2, pp. 252-258, http://ije.oxfordjournals.org/content/35/2/252.full, DOI:10.1093/ije/dyi235.

7 Elites often use the word "culture" to describe groups living in highly precarious and disturbed conditions, which is calling panfry bread a traditional food instead of something Native Americans invented after being marched to reservations and given government rations. For example, Stuart M. Butler of Brookings, and formerly the Heritage Institute, argued in the summer of 2015 in favor of "taking culture seriously" to combat what he described as widespread destitution in America. Public policy, he proceeded, should enable people to leave their neighborhoods! See: http://www.brookings.edu/blogs/social-mobility-memos/posts/2015/08/07-taking-culture-seriously-butler.

8 "Compelling evidence suggests that progressive dysfunction of the hypothalamic-pituitary-adrenal (HPA) axis, with elevated levels of circulating cortisol, is implicated in the development of visceral obesity", writes Roland Rosmond, one of the world's experts on the HPA axis. See his "Stress Induced Disturbances of the HPA Axis: A Pathway to Type 2 Diabetes?" *Medical Science Monitor,* 2003, Vol. 9:2, pp. 35-39, http://www.ncbi.nlm.nih.gov/pubmed/12601304. For the Italian study, see: Stringhini, Silvia, *et al.*, "Life-course Socioeconomic Status and DNA Methylation of Genes Regulating Inflammation", *International Journal of Epidemiology*, 2015, http://ije.oxfordjournals.org/content/early/2015/04/17/ije.dyv060.abstract, DOI: 10.1093/ije/dyv060.

9 John Calhoun in his 1962 experiment found that rats did not go forth and multiply in the large space he gave them, but created a terror regime with an 80 percent infant mortality rate, aberrant sexual behaviors, and eventual societal collapse. Perhaps aghast at how things turned out, he took to calling the asexual zombie pellet-eating rats the "beautiful ones." For an engaging review of his work, see "Crowding into the Behavioural Sink", http://www.edmondschools.net/portals/3/docs/terri_mcgill/read-crowding.pdf. Edmund Ramsden, a medical historian, recently gave a lecture arguing the rats evidently lived in an artificial environment with some spatial restrictions and so their behavior could not be associated with humans, adding: "Life in an unnatural urban environment of ever-increasing density could result in the complete devastation of humanity." Cf. http://nihrecord.nih.gov/newsletters/2008/07_25_2008/story1.htm.

10 Animals' physiological reactions to social stress vary enormously, with one Tanzanian fish even changing color in fifteen minutes upon losing territorial dominance. For some of the research reviewed here, see: Foster, Michelle T., *et al.*, "Social Defeat Increases Food Intake, Body Mass, and Adiposity In Syrian Hamsters", *American Journal of Physiology*, 2006, Vol. 209:5, pp. 1284-1293, http://ajpregu.physiology.org/content/290/5/R1284, DOI:10.1152/ajpregu.00437.2005, and Patterson, Zachary R. and Abizaid, Alfonso, "Stress Induced Obesity: Lessons from Rodent Models of Stress", *Frontiers of Neuroscience*, 2013, Vol. 7, http://www.ncbi.nlm.nih.gov/pmc/articles/PMC3721047/, DOI: 10.3389/fnins.2013.00130, and and Sanghez, V. *et al.*, "Psychosocial Stress Induces Hyperphagia and Exacerbates Diet-induced Insulin Resistance and the Manifestations of the Metabolic Syndrome", *Psychoneuroendocrinology*, 2013, Vol. 38:12, pp. 2933-2942, http://www.ncbi.nlm.nih.gov/pubmed/24060458, DOI: 10.1016/j.psyn-

euen.2013.07.022, and Maruska, Karen P. *et al.*, "Social Descent with Territory Loss Causes Rapid Behavioral, Endocrine and Transcriptional Changes in the Brain", *Journal of Experimental Biology*, 2013, Vol. 216, pp. 3656-3666, http://jeb.biologists.org/content/216/19/3656.full, DOI: 10.1242/jeb.088617.

[11] The lean season is doubly tough on chimpanzees in Uganda's Kibale National Park and elsewhere as they are known for fairly unstable hierarchies wherein dominants must always fear what we call political conspiracies. Cf. Muller, Martin N. and Wrangham, Richard W., "Dominance, Cortisol and Stress in Wild Chimpanzees", *Behavioral Ecology & Sociobiology*, 2004, Vol. 55:4, pp. 332-340, http://link.springer.com/article/10.1007/s00265-003-0713-1, DOI:10.1007/s00265-003-0713-1.

[12] When stress persists, a new and subprime homeostasis kicks in, wherein the withdrawal of comfort foods itself becomes an ulterior source of stress. Cf. Morris, Margaret J., *et al.*, "Why is Obesity Such a Problem in the 21st Century? The Intersection of Palatable Food, Cues and Reward Pathways, Stress and Cognition", *Neuroscience and Biobehavioral Reviews*, DOI: 10.1016/j.neubiorev.2014.12.002.

[13] Business, military, and government leaders attending an executive education course at Harvard University all had low salivary cortisol in a unique test of this question. They also all indicated in psychological questionnaires that they felt in control of their environments. The association between lower cortisol levels and higher social rank "is especially apparent when the hierarchy is uncontested and harassment of subordinates is frequent", noted Gary D. Shermana. See "Leadership is Associated with Lower Levels of Stress", *PNAS*, Vol. 109:44, pp. 17903-17907, http://www.pnas.org/content/109/44/17903.full, DOI: 10.1073/pnas.1207042109.

[14] Wild alpha baboons recovered 25 percent faster than others in a review of hundreds of incidents observed in Kenya's Amboseli ecosystem, where injuries outnumber illness by a factor of twelve. Biological stress indicators for them tend to have notably lower homeostatic levels but surges take them significantly higher than others. This is important, as not only does it explain why generic measurements of cortisol or other biological indicators may not map onto health reactions in a linear way at all, it also underscores how the HPA-mediated fight-or-flight stress response has a functional evolutionary rationale – it determines whether the lion catches the gazelle – and can actually augment immune function if not chronic. Stress can thus be salubrious and even a stimulant, even a "chisel of evolution", says Firdaus Dhabhar, adding that the key issue is whether the triggers activated by stress return to their baseline status or chronically persist, leading to inflammation. See his "A Hassle a Day May Keep the Pathogens Away", *Integral & Comparative Biology*, 2009, Vol. 49:3, pp. 215-236, http://icb.oxfordjournals.org/content/49/3/215.long, DOI:1 0.1093/icb/icp045. For the baboon study, see Archie, Elizabeth A., *et al.*, "Social Status Predicts Wound Healing in Wild Baboons", *PNAS*, 2012, Vol. 109:23, pp. 9017-9022, http://www.pnas.org/content/109/23/9017.full.

[15] High-ranking mandrills in Gabon have cortisol surges during the mating season, but unlike subordinates they are temporary. Females of this species inherit their rank maternally and live in matrilineal groups throughout their lives, giving them stabler biological stress profiles. Cf. Beaulieu, Michaël, *et al.*, "The Oxidative Cost of Unstable Social Dominance", *The Journal of Experimental Biology*, 2014, Vol. 217, http://jeb.biologists.org/content/217/15/2629.abstract, DOI: 10.1242/jeb.104851.

[16] Cf. Sapolsky, Robert M., "The Influence of Social Hierarchy on Primate Health", *Science*, 2005, Vol. 308, pp. 648-652, http://www.sciencemag.org/content/308/5722/648.long, DOI: 10.1126/science.1106477.

[17] Sense of coherence was a methodological concept devised by Aaron Antonovsky in 1979 in an effort to undertand why some people show greater resilience to the health risks of stress. Cf. Agardh, Emilie A., "Work Stress and Low Sense of Coherence is Associated With Type 2 Diabetes in Middle-Aged Swedish Women", *Diabetes Care*, 2003, Vol. 26:3, pp. 719-724, http://care.diabetesjournals.org/content/26/3/719.long, DOI:10.2337/diacare.26.3.719.

[18] Cf. Gimeno, David, *et al.*, "Justice at Work and Metabolic Syndrome: the Whitehall II Study", *Occupational and Environmental Medicine Journal*, 2009, Vol. 67:4, pp. 256-262, http://oem.bmj.com/content/67/4/256, DOI: 10.1136/oem.2009.047324.

[19] Tsimane are somewhat sickened by modern life. When mean village wealth measured in canoes, radios, and guns rises by the equivalent of $10, residents tend to spend an extra two days sick in bed. Cf. Von Rueden, Christopher R., *et al.*, "Political Influence Associates with Cortisol and Health Among Egalitarian Forager-Farmers", *Evolution, Medicine and Public Health*, 2014, http://www.ncbi.nlm.nih.gov/pmc/articles/PMC4178369/, DOI: 10.1093/emph/eou021, and Unduraga, Eduardo A., "Wealth Rank, Community Wealth Inequality, and Self-Reported Adult Poor Health", *Medical Anthropology Quarterly*, 2010, Vol. 24:4, pp. 522-548, http://onlinelibrary.wiley.com/doi/10.1111/j.1548-1387.2010.01121.x/full, DOI: 10.1111/j.1548-1387.2010.01121.x.

[20] Miguel Carneiro and forty other geneticists unveiled the rabbit's genome and argue that domestication came about from a host of minor genetic shifts, very few of which have been completely fixed, meaning rabbits could "rewild." See "Rabbit Genome Analysis Reveals a Polygenic Basis for Phenotypic Change During Domestication", *Science*, 2014, Vol. 345:6200, pp. 1074-1079, http://www.sciencemag.org/content/345/6200/1074.full, DOI:10.1126/science.1253714. According to the biologist and popular writer Jared Diamond, who has a beef with whoever first picked up a hoe, humans are heading in the other direction as due to our farmed diet, "the unconscious domestication of humans by agriculture that began over 10,000 years ago is still underway." See his "Evolution, Consequences and Future of Plant and Animal Domestication", *Nature*, 2002, Vol. 418:700-707, http://www.nature.com/nature/journal/v418/n6898/full/nature01019.html.

[21] Dogs, it turns out, typically present with a Type 1 diabetes-like syndrome as a result of the genetic changes that led them to separate from their wolf brethren. Cf. Osto, Melania and Lutz, Thomas A., "Translational Value of Animal Models of Obesity - Focus on Dogs And Cats", *European Journal of Pharmacology*, 2015, Vol. 759, pp. 240-252, http://www.sciencedirect.com/science/article/pii/S0014299915002526, DOI: 10.1016/j.ejphar.2015.03.036.

[22] Daniel Cossins offers a rich and wide-ranging look at how seemingly contingent social misfortune can trigger sweeping adverse biological reactions. See his "Social Adversity Shapes Humans' Immune Systems – And Probably their Susceptibility to Disease – By Altering the Expression of Large Groups of Genes", *The Scientist*, Jan. 1, 2015, http://www.the-scientist.com/?articles.view/articleNo/41708/title/Stress-Fractures/.

[23] That comfort foods – high in simple carbohydrates and fat – are instinctively sought out by the body as a way to rein in the adverse inflammatory effects of chronic stress,

essentially seeking out a metabolic negative feedback signal, was clearly articulated more than a decade ago in a way also linked to anorexia, essentially the opposite reaction to stress and more common among younger people who due to age may still have low insulin concentrations despite very high cortisol concentrations. Absent a solution to stress, tradeoff would appear to be between persistent melancholic depression and long-term health risks. Cf. Dallman, Mary F., *et al.*, "Chronic Stress and Obesity: A New View of 'Comfort Food'", *PNAS*, 2003, Vol. 100:20, pp. 11696-11701, http://www.pnas.org/content/100/20/11696.long, DOI: 10.1073/pnas.1934666100.

[24] Cf. Thurner, Stefan, "Quantification of Excess Risk for Diabetes for those Born in Times of Hunger, in an Entire Population of a Nation, Across a Century", *PNAS*, 2013, Vol. 110:12, pp. 4703-4707, http://www.pnas.org/content/110/12/4703.full, DOI:10.1073/pnas.1215626110.

[25] This maternal capital model can also fit animals. Higher-status primates, for example, have access to better food supply and can produce more and larger offspring, while their low-status brethren may face higher infant mortality and longer lactation to offset smaller sizes at birth. Cf. Wells, Jonathan C.K., "Maternal Capital and the Metabolic Ghetto: An Evolutionary Perspective on the Transgenerational Basis of Health Inequalities", *American Journal of Human Biology*, 2010, Vol. 22:1, pp. 1-17, http://onlinelibrary.wiley.com/doi/10.1002/ajhb.20994/abstract, DOI: 10.1002/ajhb.20994.

[26] India is the number two sugar producer in the world and half of the output goes to *jaggery* and *khandsari*, an unrefined white pan sugar. Cf. Singh, Suman, *et al.*, "Spoilage of Sugarcane Juice a Problem in Sugarcane Industry", *International Journal of Agricultural Engineering*, Vol. 7:1, pp. 259-263, https://www.academia.edu/7224934/Spoilage_of_sugarcane_juice-_a_problem_in_sugarcane_industry.

[27] A similar metabolic ghetto explanation may apply to African Americans, who in a different context were subject to multiple generations of malnutrition. Still today African American infants tend to be born underweight, by a full half pound compared to the US average, and high diabetes and obesity rates likely reflect a high metabolic load compared to capacity. Cf. Jasienska, G., "Low-birth Weight of Contemporary African Americans: An Intergenerational Effect of Slavery?" *American Journal of Human Biology*, 2009, Vol. 21:1, pp. 16-24, http://www.ncbi.nlm.nih.gov/pubmed/18925572, DOI:10.1002/ajhb.20824.

[28] India's large population means individual consumption of sugar is not high. Estimates vary wildly, from 18.9 kilograms a year – which would be a bit more than Japan – to an implausibly low 1.7 kilograms reported in a *Washington Post* global story using Euromonitor's data. Cf. Kaveeshwar S.A. and Cornwall, J., "The Current State of Diabetes Mellitus in India", *Australasian Medical Journal*, 2014, Vol. 7:1, pp. 45-48, http://www.ncbi.nlm.nih.gov/pmc/articles/PMC3920109/, DOI:10.4066/AMJ.2013.1979.

[29] The traditional Pima diet consisted largely of lima and tepary beans, a kind of corn with a lower glycemic index than modern American sweetcorn, and plenty of acorns, a huge human dietary source since Neolithic times. Acorns take a lot of processing work to eat but have a strong nutritional profile. Unfortunately for advocates of the view that dental caries is primarily due to sugar and was nearly absent in history, archaeologists have now unveiled definitive evidence that consumption of wild acorns led to widespread tooth decay at an early age among the Pleistocene inhabitants of what is now

Morocco some 15,000 years ago. Cf. Humphrey, Louise T., "Earliest Evidence for Caries and Exploitation of Starchy Plant Foods in Pleistocene Hunter-Gatherers from Morocco", *PNAS*, 2013, Vol. 111:3, pp. 954-959, http://www.pnas.org/content/111/3/954.full, DOI:10.1073/pnas.131817611.

30 For a detailed look at recent Pima history, see Jong, David H., *Stealing the Gila: The Pima Agricultural Economy and Water Deprivation, 1848-1921*, Arizona University Press, 2009.

31 Countless scientific papers, books and magazine articles have been written about the 20,000 or so Pima. The best, though, are by Daniel Benyshek, an anthropologist at the University of Nevada in Las Vegas, who has supplemented his social analyses with laboratory work and found that rats born to mothers who were themselves malnourished have altered insulin sensitivity regardless of diet. Cf. Benyshek, Daniel, *et al.*, " A Reconsideration of the Origins of the Type 2 Diabetes Epidemic Among Native Americans and the Implications for Intervention Policy", *Medical Anthropology: Cross-Cultural Studies in Health and Illness*, 2001, Vol. 20:1, pp. 5-64, http://www.tandfonline.com/doi/abs/10.1080/01459740.2001.9966186#.Vc8cq_mqqko, DOI: 10.1080/01459740.2001.9966186, and "Post-natal Diet Determines Insulin Resistance in Fetally Malnourished, Low Birthweight Rats (F1) but Diet does not Modify the Insulin Resistance of Their Offspring (F2)", *Life Sciences*, 2004, Vol. 74:24, pp. 3033-3041, http://www.sciencedirect.com/science/article/pii/S0024320504001468, DOI: 10.1016/j.lfs.2003.11.008.

32 The Pima's forebears living 1,000 years ago in the American Southwest ate 200 to 400 grams of fiber a day, about twenty times what Americans currently take in, according to Karl Reinhard, an archaeologist who studied ancient coprolites – fossilized fecal matter – in Antelope Cave, Arizona. The diet then consisted of the occasional rabbit and some corn along with cactus and agave, for an average glycenic index of around 23, far below the officially "low" level of 55, he says, noting that, as with the panda, it can take a lot of time to eat so much fiber. Cf. Reinhard, Karl, *et al.*, "Understanding the Pathoecological Relationship between Ancient Diet and Modern Diabetes through Coprolite Analysis: A Case Example from Antelope Cave, Mojave County, Arizona", *Papers in Natural Resources*, Paper 321, http://digitalcommons.unl.edu/cgi/viewcontent.cgi?article=1323&context=natrespapers.

33 Haven Emerson, a Columbia University professor who linked diabetes to sugar consumption, explained the malady in the 1920s as likely to afflict those "oozing with wealth, bulging with money bags, eating every day", even during wartime. More interestingly, some doctors floated the idea that Jews might be prone to diabetes because of their tendency to live in cities and their association with neurotic character typologies, which were linked in turn to acculturation syndrome after centuries of persecution. Many Jewish scholars eagerly embraced the view that they were especially prone to diabetes on the grounds that this underscored their high degree of civilization. "Diabetes enjoyed popularity as a 'Jewish' disease because science, medicine, and culture all worked together to produce believable narratives", notes Arleen Tuchman in her superb account: "Diabetes and RACE A Historical Perspective", *American Journal of Public Health*, 2011, Vol. 101:1, pp. 24-33, http://www.ncbi.nlm.nih.gov/pmc/articles/PMC3000712/, DOI: 10.2105/AJPH.2010.202564. A shift from malnutrition to abundance, coupled with cultural stress, may also explain the strikingly high diabetes incidence developed among recent arrivals in Israel from Ethiopia and Yemen.

[34] For a fine archival collation and review of these dietaries, ordered by Olin Lee Atwater and done in more than a dozen communities from Maine to New Mexico, see Robert Dirks's "Diet and Nutrition in Poor and Minority Communities in the United States 100 Years Ago", *Annual Review of Nutrition*, 2003, vol. 23, pp. 81-100, http://www.annualreviews.org/doi/abs/10.1146/annurev.nutr.23.011702.073341.

[35] It's not clear whether or how this phenotype might be modified by social mobility over the life course. The researchers note it's possible that inflammatory responsivity might dampen amid affluence, but it's not clear whether that would have positive or negative consequences for health down the road. Cf. Millera, Gregory E., *et al.*, "Low Early-life Social Class Leaves a Biological Residue Manifested by Decreased Glucocorticoid and Increased Pro-inflammatory Signaling", *PNAS*, Vol. 106:34, pp. 14716-14721, http://www.pnas.org/content/106/34/14716.full, DOI: 10.1073/pnas.0902971106.

[36] In a pure correlation study based on 644 people that did not consider diet – having no reason to assume great differences – poor housing, and not neighborhood conditions or noise levels, appeared as an independent contributor to the risk of diabetes in urban, middle-aged African-Americans. Cf. Schootman, Mario, "The Effect of Adverse Housing and Neighborhood Conditions on the Development of Diabetes Mellitus among Middle-aged African-Americans", *American Journal of Epidemiology*, 2007, Vol. 166:4, pp. 379-387, http://aje.oxfordjournals.org/content/166/4/379.abstract, DOI: 10.1093/aje/kwm190. For the Manhattan study, see Wallace, Deborah, "Community Stress, Demoralization and Body Mass Index: Evidence for Social Signal Transduction", *Social Science & Medicine*, 2003, Vol. 56:12, pp. 2467-2478, http://www.ncbi.nlm.nih.gov/pubmed/12742610.

[37] Cf. Poulter, N.R., "The Kenyan Luo Mmigration Sstudy", *British Medical Journal*, 1990, Vol. 300, pp. 967-972, http://www.ncbi.nlm.nih.gov/pmc/articles/PMC1662695/, and Unwin, N., "Changes In Blood Pressure and Lipids Associated with Rural to Urban Migration in Tanzania", *Journal of Human Hypertension*, 2006, Vol. 20, pp. 704-706, http://www.nature.com/jhh/journal/v20/n9/full/1002056a.html, DOI: 10.1038/sj.jhh.1002056, and Kinra, Sanjay, *et al.*, "Association Between Urban Life-Years and Cardiometabolic Risk: The Indian Migration Study", *American Journal of Epidemiology*, 2011, http://aje.oxfordjournals.org/content/early/2011/05/27/aje.kwr053.full, DOI: 10.1093/aje/kwr053, and Fang, Carolyn Y., *et al.*, "Stressful Life Events are Associated with Insulin Resistance Among Chinese Immigrant Women in The United States", *Preventive Medicine Reports*, 2015, Vol. 2, pp. 563-567, http://www.sciencedirect.com/science/article/pii/S2211335515000856, DOI:10.1016/j.pmedr.2015.06.013.

[38] The number of Americans who live in communities where the poverty rate is above 40 percent, which impacts local consumption options, has nearly doubled since 2000 to 14 million. Increasingly these neighborhoods are in close-in suburbs of midsized cities. Cf. Semuels, Alana, "The Resurrection of America's Slums", *The Atlantic*, Aug. 9, 2015, http://www.theatlantic.com/business/archive/2015/08/more-americans-are-living-in-slums/400832/.

[39] Cf. Nord, Mark, "Food Spending Declined and Food Insecurity Increased for Middle-income and Low-income Households from 2000 to 2007", *USDA Economic Information Bulletin*, Oct. 2009, http://www.ers.usda.gov/publications/eib-economic-information-bulletin/eib61.aspx. USDA's latest update on food insecurity is here: http://

www.ers.usda.gov/topics/food-nutrition-assistance/food-security-in-the-us/key-statistics-graphics.aspx#verylow.

[40] The English pattern may still exist. Among a large sample of Hertsfordshire men born around 1930, those with low birth weight were three times more likely to be diabetic by age 65 than those with robust birth weights. "The associations between birth weight and later glucose tolerance are independent of adult lifestyle influences", although obesity exacerbates the risks for a body with reduced ability to make insulin, noted David Barker, who is one of the avatars of theories about fetal nutrition. Cf. Godfrey, K.M. and Barker, D.J., "Fetal Nutrition and Adult Disease", *American Journal of Clinical Nutrition,* 2000, Vol. 71:5, pp. 1344-1352, http://www.ncbi.nlm.nih.gov/pubmed/10799412. Regarding historical height, England was just the pinnacle of a European trend, as German nobility were also better able to commandeer adequate nutrients and so towered over their servants. Cf. Komlos, John H., "On English Pygmies and Giants: the Physical Stature of English Youth in the late-18th and early-19th Centuries", University of Munich Discussion Paper, 2005, http://epub.ub.uni-muenchen.de/573/1/ch.

[41] Data for almost 70,000 Canadians in Ontario province showed that health care costs including hospital care, emergency department visits, physician services, and home-care services as well as prescription drugs rose 121 percent for households facing severe food insecurity and 23 percent for those facing the mildest form of privation. In Canada, where food insecurity levels are broadly similar to the USA, average additional health care costs faced by food-insecure families was equal to the per capita cost of diabetes treatment in Canada. Cf. Tarasuk, Valerie, "Association Between Household Food Insecurity and Annual Health Care Costs", *Canadian Medical Association Journal,* 2015, http://www.cmaj.ca/content/early/2015/08/10/cmaj.150234, DOI: 10.1503/cmaj.150234.

[42] While official US figures for the working-age poverty rate have remained close to 10 percent over the past fifty years, a breakout of the data show that the prospects for spending some time in acute poverty grew sharply, at times doubling, for people in their twenties, thirties, and forties, with a big spike occurring in the 1990s. A new study suggests more than four out of ten American 40-year-olds will live in a household facing extreme poverty for at least a year, with the most notable increase taking place at an age associated with having young children living at home. Cf. Rank, Mark R. and Hirschl, Thomas A., "The Likelihood of Experiencing Relative Poverty over the Life Course", *Plos,* 2015, http://journals.plos.org/plosone/article?id=10.1371/journal.pone.0133513, DOI:10.1371/journal.pone.0133513, and Sandoval, Daniel A., *et al.,* "The Increasing Risk of Poverty Across the American Life Couse", *Demography,* 2009, Vol. 46:4, pp. 717-737, http://www.ncbi.nlm.nih.gov/pmc/articles/PMC2831356/.

[43] Of course, declining soda sales may simply mean booming sales of rival drinks like Snapple, which is sweetened but not carbonated, energy drinks which often have more sugar than the big branded colas, or bottled water, which is poised to overtake carbonated drinks in terms of value by 2017. Cf. Suddath, Clare and Stanford, Duane,

"Coke Confronts its Big Fat Problem", *Bloomberg Business Week*, July 31, 2014, http://www.bloomberg.com/bw/articles/2014-07-31/coca-cola-sales-decline-health-concerns-spur-relaunch.

44 The data, presented without the generational lag come from Gross, Lee S., *et al.*, "Increased Consumption of Refined Carbohydrates and the Epidemic of Type 2 Diabetes in the United States: An Ecologic Assessment", *American Journal of Clinical Nutrition*", 2004, Vol. 79:5, pp. 774-779, http://ajcn.nutrition.org/content/79/5/774.full.

45 One reason why a cure for metabolic syndrome has proven so elusive, and requires a regular rotation of culprits, is that its markers are mistaken for causes, Anne-Thea McGill says in a fascinating paper that strongly argues for the evolutionary importance of the microbiome in allocation energy to brain and body and sees the energy balance and dietary claims to resolve obesity as symptoms of disorder. Humans are unusual in having outsourced some of their metabolic enzymes, so we need external inputs such as vitamin C. While that was done to make brain development more efficient, the tradeoff was a shorter intestine, and so we require external inputs from micro- and phyto-nutrients that gut microbes know how to use. Microbes also detoxify xenobiotics or toxins that nomadic foragers inevitably eat. Without being fed or stimulated, this anti-oxidizing and immune-boosting system atrophies, and the *Firmicutes* bacteria multiply. See McGill, Anne-Thea, "Causes of Metabolic Syndrome and Obesity-related Co-morbidities Part 1: A Composite Unifying Theory Review of Human-specific Co-adaptations to Brain Energy Consumption", *Archives of Public Health*, 2014, Vol. 72:1, http://www.ncbi.nlm.nih.gov/pmc/articles/PMC4335398/, DOI: 10.1186/2049-3258-72-30.

46 As this study used self-reported dietaries, analysts double-checked for weight bias and found that heavier kids were indeed most likely to lowball what they ate. However, whites were 50 percent more likely than South Asians to do this. Cf. Donin, A.S., *et al.*, "Nutritional Composition of the Diets of South Asian, Black African-Caribbean and White European Children in the United Kingdom", *British Journal of Nutrition*, 2010, Vol. 104, pp. 276-285, http://journals.cambridge.org/action/displayFulltext?type=6&fid=7835468&jid=BJN&volumeId=104&issueId=02&aid=7835467&bodyId=&membershipNumber=&societyETOCSession=&fulltextType=RA&fileId=S000711451000070X, DOI: 10.1017/S007114510000070X.

47 Norwegian scholars looking at how South Asians are faring around Europe cogently noted that acculturation may be a shock because immigrants identify convenience foods with the local cultural diet, a notion cynics may wink at but is not, at least yet, true! Indeed, this research garnered a headline declaring "Nordic Foods Make Immigrants Sick!" Cf. Holmboe-Ottesen, Gerd and Wandel, Margereta, "Changes in Dietary Habits After Migration and Consequences for Health: A focus on South Asians in Europe", *Food & Nutrition Research*, 2012, Vol. 56 http://www.ncbi.nlm.nih.gov/pmc/articles/PMC3492807/, DOI: 10.3402/fnr.v56i0.18891.

Chapter 7

1 From the report on the typhus epidemic in Upper Silesia in 1848, when a tenth of the population died in abject poverty. The founder of German social medicine described it as a failure of the Prussian state and fixable only with "full and unlimited democracy" for the local Polish-speaking population. See Taylor, Rex and Rieger, Annelie, "Rudolf Virchow on the Typhus Epidemic in Upper Silesia: An Introduction and Translation", *Sociology of Health and Illness*, 1984, Vol. 6:2, pp. 201-217, http://onlinelibrary.wiley.com/doi/10.1111/1467-9566.ep10778374/pdf.

2 USDA economists say fresh produce prices have moved broadly in tandem with snack foods, with both posting secular declines in inflation-adjusted terms. However, that argument is based on the new trend for pre-cut and pre-washed items, which is a shopping convenience. Insofar as they boost consumption of dietary fibers that innovation is welcome; however, its benefits are likely accrue only to the more affluent households who are not cutting back their spending on food. Cf. Kuchler, Fred and Stewart, Hayden, "Price Trends are Similar for Fruits, Vegetables, and Snack Foods", *USDA Economic Research Service Report No. 55*, 2008, http://www.ers.usda.gov/media/224301/err55.pdf.

3 The energy content of a potato chip, measured in terms of weight, is up to 60 times higher than a vegetable, making a mockery of claims that adequate diets are within the reach of all and the poor need simply to be educated. Cf. Drewnowski, Adam, "The Real Contribution of Added Sugars and Fats to Obesity", *Epidemiology Review*, 2007, Vol. 29:1, pp. 160-171, http://epirev.oxfordjournals.org/content/29/1/160.full DOI: 10.1093/epirev/mxm011.

4 A similar logic may apply to the obesity pattern in developing countries, as typically it is highest among the affluent. Some World Bank officials once argued that public health resources in such countries should focus on infectious diseases afflicting the poor, but others say obesity and diabetes should be made a priority immediately as while the affluent will benefit initially, an inflection point is looming. One study aggregating global data found that mean BMI peaks when national annual incomes reach the equivalent in purchasing power of $12,500 for women and $17,000 for men. Women's average BMI then begins to drop in all countries except the USA although its outlier status in this regard may disappear when social class is factored in. See Ezzati, Majid, *et al.*, "Rethinking the 'Diseases of Affluence' Paradigm: Global Patterns of Nutritional Risks in Relation to Economic Development", *Plos*, 2005, http://journals.plos.org/plosmedicine/article?id=10.1371/journal.pmed.0020133, DOI: 10.1371/journal.pmed.0020133. For a close look at France, see a report from the government's nutrition surveillance unit: http://www.ncbi.nlm.nih.gov/pubmed/20497773.

5 Drewnowski himself tested the economic viability of procuring a Mediterranean diet in Seattle and found that it would require slashing back on fish and leafy greens and doubling down on legumes and beans. Cf. Drewnowski, Adam and Eichelsdoerfer, Petra, "The Mediterranean Diet: Does it Have to Cost More?" *Public Health and Nutrition*, 2009, Vol. 12:9, pp. 1621-1628, http://www.ncbi.nlm.nih.gov/pmc/articles/PMC2849996/, DOI: 10.1017/S1368980009990462. For the Spanish study, see: Lopez, C.N., *et al.*, "Costs of Mediterranean and Western Dietary Patterns in a Spanish Cohort and their Relationship

with Prospective Weight Change", *Journal of Epidemiology and Community Health*, 2009, Vol. 63:11, pp. 920-927, http://www.ncbi.nlm.nih.gov/pubmed/19762456. Another analysis from Spain, covering a broader social sample, reached a similar monetary conclusion. Its authors noted that fewer than one in four households adhered to the Mediterranean diet and suggested that slashing the prices of its main components by 50 percent might be required to increase consumption. Cf. Schröder, H., *et al.*, "High Monetary Costs of Dietary Patterns Associated with Lower Body Mass Index: A Population-Based Study", *International Journal of Obesity*, 2006, Vol. 30, pp. 1574-1479, http://www.nature.com/ijo/journal/v30/n10/full/0803308a.html, DOI: 10.1038/sj.ijo.0803308. For US food budgets, see the USDA's data at: http://www.ers.usda.gov/data-products/ag-and-food-statistics-charting-the-essentials/food-prices-and-spending.aspx.

[6] Cf. Wiggins, Steve, *et al.*, "The Rising Cost of a Healthy diet", ODI, 2015, http://www.odi.org/sites/odi.org.uk/files/odi-assets/publications-opinion-files/9580.pdf.

[7] Popkin was actually cited as saying Chinese eat 300 to 400 grams of oils a day, a level twenty times higher than recommended by the American Heart Association. Presumably he said or meant calories, in which case the level is only two or three times higher. Cf. Levitt, Tom, "China Facing Bigger Dietary Health Crisis than the US", *China Dialogue*, July 4, 2014, https://www.chinadialogue.net/article/show/single/en/6880-China-facing-bigger-dietary-health-crisis-than-the-US.

[8] The chubbier Chinese kids also felt they were healthier than others. It's worth remembering that their grandparents lived through one of the most severe famines in world history. Cf, Hsu, Ya-Wen, *et al.*, "Correlates of Overweight Status in Chinese Youth: An East-West Paradox", *American Journal of Health Behavior*, 2011, Vol. 35:4, pp. 496-506, http://www.ncbi.nlm.nih.gov/pubmed/22040595. Median consumption of oils in China was 42 grams according to this study, done by researchers from Australia, Norway, Finland, and China. Cf. Shi, Z., et al, "Vegetable-rich Food Pattern is Related to Obesity in China", *International Journal of Obesity*, 2008, Vol. 32, pp. 975-984, http://www.nature.com/ijo/journal/v32/n6/abs/ijo200821a.html DOI: 10.1038/ijo.2008.21.

[9] A detailed government analysis of consumption patterns also noted that adolescent males are huge if temporary sugar consumers, with those aged 12-30 taking in 40 percent more than the average for all men and almost twice the level of all women. Cf. Haley, Stephen, *et al.*, "Sweetener Consumption in the United States: Distribution by Demographic and Product Characteristics", USDA Economic Research Service, 2005, http://www.ers.usda.gov/media/326278/sss24301_002.pdf.

[10] For the European studies, see: Irala-Estévez, J.D., *et al.*, "A Systematic Review of Socio-Economic Differences in Food Habits in Europe: Consumption of Fruit and Vegetables", *European Journal of Clinical Nutrition*, 2000, Vol. 54:9, pp. 706-14, http://www.ncbi.nlm.nih.gov/pubmed/11002383 and Perrin, A.E., *et al.*, "Ten-year Trends of Dietary Intake in a Middle-aged French Population: Relationship with Educational Level", *European Journal of Clinical Nutrition*, Vol. 56:5, pp. 393-401, http://www.nature.com/ejcn/journal/v56/n5/full/1601322a.html. For the British study, see Scientific Advisory Committee on Nutrition, 2014, *Draft Consultation Report*, p.21, https://www.gov.uk/government/uploads/system/uploads/attachment_data/file/339771/Draft_SACN_Carbohydrates_and_Health_report_consultation.pdf.

[11] Monaghan's six types of obesity epidemic entrepreneurs engage in activities ranging from ostensibly neutral science to paternalistic and potentially lucrative advisory services – he names Philip James, chair of the International Obesity Task force and advisor to the WHO – and ultimately the "entrepreneurial self" who joins a fitness center and buys custom pharmaceuticals or a home video game that measures their BMI. "Politically, the stage is set for an ongoing pernicious power play, which may be sugar-coated with appeals to health and a 'care of the self' ethic, but which will have many 'big losers'..." Cf. Monaghan, Lee F., "Obesity Epidemic Entrepreneurs: Types, Practices and Interests", *Body & Society*, 2010, Vol. 16:2, pp. 37-71, http://bod.sagepub.com/content/16/2/37.short, DOI:10.1177/1357034X10364769.

[12] The hot topic for the US guidelines is meat, as the advisory committee suggested less should be eaten on environmental grounds. See http://www.health.gov/dietaryguidelines/2015-scientific-report/PDFs/Scientific-Report-of-the-2015-Dietary-Guidelines-Advisory-Committee.pdf.

[13] Interestingly SACN noted that evidence for a link between sugar-sweetened beverages and BMI was based entirely on US studies, whereas the Europe-based studies it consulted found no relation. Cf. "Carbohydrates and Health", SACN, 2015, https://www.gov.uk/government/uploads/system/uploads/attachment_data/file/445503/SACN_Carbohydrates_and_Health.pdf.

[14] Cf. Blair, Steven N., "Energy Balance: A Crucial Issue for Exercise and Sports medicine", *British Journal of Sports Medicine*, 2015, http://bjsm.bmj.com/content/early/2015/04/16/bjsports-2015-094592, DOI: 10.1136/bjsports-2015-094592.full. For The Times story, see O'Connor, Anahad, "Coca-Cola Funds Scientists Who Shift Blame for Obesity Away From Bad Diets", *The New York Times*, Aug. 9, 2015, http://well.blogs.nytimes.com/2015/08/09/coca-cola-funds-scientists-who-shift-blame-for-obesity-away-from-bad-diets/?_r=0.

[15] Coca-Cola's glycemic index is between 63 and 90 according to various studies. Pure glucose is 100, as is white bread. The glycemic load is a function of typical serving size. The SACN found the glycemic index had no clinical relevance, but for a recent classification of foods from the Harvard Medical School, see this website: http://www.health.harvard.edu/healthy-eating/glycemic_index_and_glycemic_load_for_100_foods.

[16] Cf. Malhotra, A., *et al.*, "It is Time to Bust the Myth of Physical Inactivity and Obesity: You Cannot Outrun a Bad Diet", *British Journal of Sports Medicine*, 2015, http://bjsm.bmj.com/content/early/2015/05/07/bjsports-2015-094911.full, DOI: 10.1136/bjsports-2015-09491. Britain's chief medical officer reported in 2009 that physical activity can lower diabetes risk by 50 percent. See http://www.sthc.co.uk/Documents/CMO_Report_2009.pdf.

[17] The study is hard to assess as it reported that the mean energy intake per day was around 1,600 calories, an extraordinarily low amount given the average BMI for participants was above 29. The mean level reflected remarkable variation in self-reported energy intakes, which for women ranged from under 600 calories a day to above 4,000! Cf. McTiernen, Anne, *et al.*, "Exercise Effect on Weight and Body Fat in Men and Women", *Obesity*, 2007, Vol. 15:6, pp. 1496-1512, http://onlinelibrary.wiley.com/doi/10.1038/oby.2007.178/full, DOI: 10.1038/oby.2007.178. The cited study is hardly alone in struggling with unreliable data. Professor Blair, one of the recipients of Coca-Cola's funding, notes that data from nine NHANES surveys, the US benchmark

database, found that Americans should have lost 32 kilograms in the 1970s and then gained 98 kilograms from 1988 to 2010! His paper is posted on the GERB website of all places. See https://gebn.org/asset/articles/Causes_of_world-wide_inc_in_BW-Shook-US_Endochronology-June.pdf.

18 Apart from the stage antics, the Malhotra vs. Blair dispute hangs on whether exercise is offset by extra caloric intake. Simply put, weight loss does not track rising or falling energy consumption in a linear way because the body adjusts its metabolism accordingly. A new high-powered model of how the energy imbalance works finds that Americans today need an additional 220 calories a day compared to 1975 due to weight gains since then. As actual consumption is 180 calories higher, the rest must be reduced energy expenditure. However, losing fat tissue takes five times more of an adjustment than losing lean tissue, so exercisers who manage to convert some of the former to the latter may not lose much weight but have markedly changed their prospects for doing so. While enticed by the theoretical idea that dietary composition may impact weight dynamics, particularly regarding protein, the authors calculate that a shift from carbohydrates to fat would produce only marginal results, concluding that the old adage that "a calorie is a calorie" remains a practical rule of thumb. Cf. Hall, Kevin, D., *et al.*, "Quantification of Energy Imbalance on Bodyweight", *The Lancet*, 2014, Vol. 378, http://www.ncbi.nlm.nih.gv/pmc/articles/PMC3880593/ DOI: 10.1016/S0140-6736(11)60812-X.

19 Cf. Asby, Daniel J., *et al.*, "AMPK Activation via Modulation of De Novo Purine Biosynthesis with an Inhibitor of ATIC Homodimerization", *Chemistry & Biology*, Vol. 22:7, pp. 838-848, http://www.sciencedirect.com/science/article/pii/S1074552115002343, DOI: 10.1016/j.chembiol.2015.06.008. For the study of energy spent on the job, see: Church, T.S., *et al.*, "Trends over 5 Decades in U.S. Occupation-Related Physical Activity and Their Associations with Obesity", *Plos ONE*, 2011, Vol. 6:5, http://journals.plos.org/plosone/article?id=10.1371/journal.pone.0019657, DOI:10.1371/journal.pone.0019657.

20 Lars Thorup Larsen has a fascinating angle on the evolution of US and European public health discourses in recent decades. Americans, he notes, like to use optimistic language and talk of "great progress" even when actual achievements have no evident link to the agenda. The style in his native Denmark is more self-critical and catastrophic in its retrospective preambles, but still ends up celebrating improvements on preventive methods that haven't been shown to be particularly successful. See his "Is Prevention Better than Cure? Public Health Policy and the Circular Structure of Learning", *American Political Science Association Annual Meeting Paper*, 2010, http://papers.ssrn.com/sol3/papers.cfm?abstract_id=1642354.

21 Cf. For the government blueprint, see http://www.healthypeople.gov/, and for the review, see *Healthy People 2010 Final Review*, Centers for Disease Control and Prevention, 2013, http://www.cdc.gov/nchs/healthy_people/hp2010/hp2010_final_review.htm.

22 The WHO recommends less than 2,000 milligrams of sodium and at least 3,510 milligrams of potassium per person per day. Drewnowski calculated that the difference in diet costs between those with the highest and lowest potassium intakes is $1.49 a day, essentially the same as the difference in the food budget between an affluent and a poor person. See his "The Feasibility of Meeting the WHO Guidelines for Sodium and Potassium: A Cross-national Comparison Study", *BMJ Open*, 2015, Vol. 5, http://bmjopen.

bmj.com/content/5/3/e006625.full, DOI:10.1136/bmjopen-2014-006625. For the USDA study on vegetables, see Guthrie, Joanne and Biing-Hwan Lin, "Healthy Vegetables Undermined by the Company they Keep", USDA Economic Research Service, 2014, http://www.ers.usda.gov/amber-waves/2014-may/healthy-vegetables-undermined-by-the-company-they-keep.aspx#.VX2KJPmqqko.

[23] Potassium deficiency is often noted to be of clinical relevance in diabetes patients, so commandeering or subsidizing such foods for distribution to populations at risk would fit well into a public policy aimed at tackling obesity and curbing future health care costs. Cf. Chatterjee, Ranee, *et al.*, "Potassium and Risk of Type 2 Diabetes", *Expert Review of Endocrinology & Metabolism*, 2011, Vol. 6:5, pp. 665-672, http://www.ncbi.nlm.nih.gov/pmc/articles/PMC3197792/ DOI:10.1586/eem.11.60.

Chapter 8

1 The lead author of the poll cited went on to do another which concluded that associating companies with lobbying, marketing tactics aimed at children, and product manipulation would bolster support for public measures against soda companies. Here's the very well-executed main analysis: Barry, C.L., et al, "Obesity Metaphors: How Beliefs about the Causes of Obesity Affect Support for Public Policy", *Milbank Quarterly*, 2009, Vol. 87:1, pp. 7-47, http://www.ncbi.nlm.nih.gov/pmc/articles/PMC2879183/, DOI: 10.1111/j.1468-0009.2009.00546.x.

2 News stories often also say that revenue from the tax would be used to improve public health. Once in hand, politicians may of course be enticed to use them differently, as when a Los Angeles mayor proposed using funds from the tobacco settlement to pay court-awarded damages to victims of violence by police offers. Cf. Niederdeppe, Jeff, "News Coverage of Sugar-sweetened Beverage Taxes: Pro- and Antitax Arguments in Public Discourse", *American Journal of Public Health*, 2013, Vol. 103:6, pp. 92-98, http://www.ncbi.nlm.nih.gov/pmc/articles/PMC3698716/, DOI: 10.2105/AJPH.2012.301023.

3 In a highly-documented study, biologist Milind Watve and colleagues in Pune, India, suggest that oxidative stress, which damages tissue critical to metabolic processes, stems from a redistribution of immunological resources accompanying a non-injury-prone lifestyle they identify as that of the "citizen" rather than the "soldier." This echoes with the common finding that diabetic rats have weak spatial agility but strong memory skills. They hope their insight will lead to efforts to move beyond current diabetic therapies designed to manage the disease rather than aspire to cure it. Cf. Belsare, Prajakta, *et al.*, "Metabolic Syndrome: Aggression Control Mechanisms Gone out of Control", *Medical Hypotheses*, 2010, Vol. 74, pp. 578-589, http://www.ncbi.nlm.nih.gov/pubmed/19800745, DOI:10.1016/j.mehy.2009.09.014.

4 Cf. Unger, Roger H. and Scherer, Philipp E., "Gluttony, Sloth and the Metabolic Syndrome: A Roadmap to Lipotoxicity", *Trends in Endocrinoogy & Metabolism*, 2010, Vol. 21:6, pp. 345-352, DOI:10.1016/j.temp.2010.01.009.

5 Cf. Chaput, J.-P., *et al.*, "Obesity: A Disease or a Biological Adaptation?" *Obesity Reviews*, 2012, Vol. 13:8, pp. 681-691, http://onlinelibrary.wiley.com/doi/10.1111/j.1467-789X.2012.00992.x/full, DOI:10.1111/j.1467-789X.2012.00992.x.

6 France's development of its *appelations d'origine* was born as a form of self-regulation in the food and drinks sector, in contrast to the UK's efforts to set rules. The vested interests behind such differences vary between countries and over time; British milk rules demanded that milk be sold "as it came from the cow" and would until 2008 formally have considered illegal milk produced in Denmark, where it was routine for the huge dairy industry to extract the creamiest bit to make butter. Cf. Atkins, Peter J., "The Material Histories of Food Quality and Composition", *Endeavour*, 2011, Vol. 2-3, http://www.ncbi.nlm.nih.gov/pubmed/21924495. For the parliamentary report, see "Atti della giunta per la Inchesta Agraria e sulle condizione della classe agricola", edited by Jacini, Stefano, 1885, https://archive.org/stream/attidellagiunta00jacigoog#page/n4/mode/2up.

7 Gong, Fayong, *et al.*, "Hypoglycemic Effects of Crude Polysaccharide from Purslane", *International Journal of Molecular Science*, 2009, Vol. 10:3, pp. 880-888, http://www.ncbi.nlm.nih.gov/pmc/articles/PMC2672007/, DOI:10.3390/ijms10030880.

[8] For a deeper look at what made the Mediterranean diet tick, see Simopoulos, Artemis P., "The Mediterranean Diet: What is so Special about the Diet of Greece? The Scientific Evidence", *Journal of Nutrition*, 2001, Vol. 1:131, pp. 3065-3073, http://www.ncbi.nlm.nih.gov/pubmed/11694649. For current obesity data, see Vardavas, C.I., *et al.*, "Prevalence of Obesity and Physical Inactivity Among Farmers from Crete", *Nutrition, Metabolism & Cardiovascular Diseases*, 2009, Vol. 19, pp. 156-162. For a forty-year survey of food trends, see Noah, A. and Truswell, S. "Commodities Consumed in Italy, Greece and Other Mediterranean Countries Compared with Australia in the 1960s and 1990s", *Asia Pacific Journal of Clinical Nutrition*, 2003, Vol. 12:1, pp. 23-29, http://www.ncbi.nlm.nih.gov/pubmed/12737007. For a deep technical dive into purslane, see Gonnella, Maria, *et al.*, "Purslane: A Review of its Potential for Health and Agricultural Aspects", *The European Journal of Plant Science and Biotechnology*, 2010, Vol. 4:1, pp. 131-136, http://www.researchgate.net/publication/256547185_Purslane_A_Review_of_its_Potential_for_Health_and_Agricultural_Aspects.

[9] Gary Paul Nabhan quotes several people saying this in a chapter on Crete in his 2004 book on place-based diets, *Food, Genes and Culture: Eating Right for Your Origins*, and it emerges in both the data and the pretext of a 2012 paper by Antonia Psaradouki and colleagues, who are keen to revive the knowledge needed to identify the plants. See "Ten Indigenous Edible Plants: Contemporary Use in Eastern Crete, Greece", *Culture, Agriculture, Food and Environment*, Vol. 34:2, pp.172-177, http://onlinelibrary.wiley.com/doi/10.1111/j.2153-9561.2012.01076.x/abstract 10.1111/j.2153-9561.2012.01076.x.

[10] A new doctoral dissertation in Italy explored ways the confectionery sector can recapture sugar cane's bioactive micronutrients and made an experimental gelato using molasses. See Valli, Veronica, "Possibilities for the Healthy and Nutritional Improvement of Confectionery and Sweet Products", University of Bologna, 2014, http://amsdottorato.unibo.it/6359/1/Valli_Veronica_tesi.pdf. For a review of sugar cane's phytochemical profile, see Singh, Amandeep, *et al.*, "Phytochemical Profile of Sugarcane and its Potential Health Aspects", *Pharmacognosy Review*, 2015, Vol. 9:17, pp. 45-54, http://www.ncbi.nlm.nih.gov/pmc/articles/PMC4441162/, DOI: 10.4103/0973-7847.156340. For a review of non-centrifugal cane sugar's 14 key minerals and 13 vitamins as well as phenolics, amino acids and oligosaccharides, see Jaffe, Walter R., "Nutritional and Functional Components of Non-centrifugal Cane Sugar: A Compilation of the Data from the Analytical Literature", *Journal of Food Composition and Analysis*, 2015, Vol. 43, pp.194-202, http://www.sciencedirect.com/science/article/pii/S0889157515001490, DOI: 10.1016/j.jfca.2015.06.007.

[11] The huge success of cup holders in the 1980s probably contributed to the social acceptance of eating and drinking throughout the day and foods designed for that, making it one of many culprits of weight gain, according to David Klurfeld, a USDA economist, who adds: "reasonable response to overconsumption by a fraction of the population is not to prescribe zero intake by anyone. Moderation is a concept that does not resonate with consumers or most scientists." See his "What do Government Agencies Consider in the Debate Over Added Sugars?" *Advances in Nutrition*, 2012, Vol. 4:2, pp. 257-261, http://www.ncbi.nlm.nih.gov/pmc/articles/PMC3649106/, DOI: 10.3945/an.112.003004.

[12] Actual risk factors are likely to be higher as workers experiencing illness are presumably more likely to quit. For the Belgian study, see de De Bacquer, D., *et al.*, "Rotating Shift Work and the Metabolic Syndrome", *International Journal of Epidemiolo-*

gy, 2009, Vol. 38:3, pp. 848-854, http://ije.oxfordjournals.org/content/38/3/848.full, DOI:10.1093/ije/dyn360. For the Japan study, see Ika, K., *et al.*, "Shift Work and Diabetes Mellitus Among Male Workers in Japan", *Acta Med Okayama*, 2013, Vol. 67:1, pp. 25-33, http://www.ncbi.nlm.nih.gov/pubmed/23439506?dopt=Abstract. For the Italian study, see Di Lorenzo, L., *et al.*, "Effect of Shift Work on Body Mass Index", *International Journal of Obesity*, 2003, Vol. 27, pp. 1353-1358, http://www.nature.com/ijo/journal/v27/n11/full/0802419a.html, DOI:10.1038/sj.ijo.0802419.

[13] Cf. Calvin, Andrew D., *et al.*, "Effects of Experimental Sleep Restriction on Caloric Intake and Activity Energy Expenditure", *Chest*, 2013, Vol. 144:1, pp. 79-86, http://www.ncbi.nlm.nih.gov/pmc/articles/PMC3707179/, DOI:10.1378/chest.12-2829.

[14] A previous study on young and slim adults in Chicago found activation of the HPA axis led to a 16 percent drop in total insulin sensitivity among volunteers after four days of only 4.5 hours of sleep, and with twice as sharp a drop in adipose tissue. Cf. Broussard, Josiane, L., *et al.*, "Impaired Insulin Signaling in Human Adipocytes After Experimental Sleep Restriction", *Annals of Internal Medicine*, 2012, Vol. 157:8, pp. 549-557, http://www.ncbi.nlm.nih.gov/pmc/articles/PMC4435718/, DOI: 10.7326/0003-4819-157-8-201210160-00005. For the Swedish study, see Cedernaes, Jonathan, *et al.*, "Acute Sleep Loss Induces Tissue-specific Epigenetic and Transcriptional Alterations to Circadian Clock Genes in Men", *The Journal of Clinical Endocrinology & Metabolism*, 2015, http://press.endocrine.org/doi/pdf/10.1210/JC.2015-2284, DOI:10.1210/JC.2015-2284. The sleep deficit data come from Gallup, see http://www.gallup.com/poll/166553/less-recommended-amount-sleep.aspx.

[15] The CDC noted that 6.5 percent of Americans aged 25 to 45 – the generation that came of age as sugar consumption and obesity began to decline and media stories about them as a public health epidemic began to surge – admitted that they had fallen asleep while driving in the past month. See http://www.cdc.gov/features/dssleep/.

[16] Brazil's dietary guidelines, which are a model for their clear language, actually do urge eating in common, even calling it an evolutionary achievement. See: http://www.fao.org/nutrition/education/food-dietary-guidelines/regions/brazil/en/. For a review of mostly US research on family meals, see http://www.human.cornell.edu/pam/outreach/upload/Family-Mealtimes-2.pdf.

[17] In a deal brokered in 2014 by the Clinton Global Initiative, the three biggest soda companies pledged to cut by a fifth the per capita beverage calories in the US by 2025 through marketing, distribution and packaging initiatives.

[18] "Children give great prestige to foods that adults will not eat", according to a superb ethnography of fifth-grade kids in Oregon and their school lunches by Andrea Thompson. Foods with strange colors and anomalous sizes were particularly appreciated as cool, and so were foods allowing "self-agency" such as microwavable snacks. Energy drinks were used as a form of social capital, she found. Echoing the junk-food smuggling in British schools, she found that many of her 11-year-old informants engaged in brisk contraband trade of "energy pills", easily available at local shops. All the kids agreed that school lunches, provided by Sodexho, a French multinational with global sales only slightly below those of McDonald's, were awful, served "only to make money", and failed to meet any of the nutritional claims made by the public school that

served them. "Americans tend to approach societal problems by asking what policies can we make, what rules can we put in place, and how can we control the situation", Thompson observes. "This line of question is not creating change." See her "'I AM COLD LUNCH': An Anthropological Perspective on Children's Cultural Identity and Understanding of Food through an Ethnographic Study of Food and Eating in Public Elementary Schools", BA thesis, Pacific University, 2007, http://commons.pacificu.edu/cassoc/3/.

19 Before championing public sanitation works, Edmund Chadwick was the administrator of Britain's Poor Law and aggressively shot down any suggestion that people were dying of hunger, insisting instead that deaths be registered as due to a specific disease. Such "ontological" definitions dissuaded health practitioners from focusing on the political and living conditions of people who were disproportionately affected by the infectious diseases of the time. Cf. Hamlin, Christopher, "Could You Starve to Death in England in 1839? The Chadwick-Farr Controversy and the Loss of the 'Social' in Public Health", *American Journal of Public Health*, 1995, Vol. 85:6, pp. 856-866, http://www.ncbi.nlm.nih.gov/pmc/articles/PMC1615507/.

20 It took a century and two world wars for the region to become part of Poland. Virchow, who later protested Bismarck's welfare reforms on the grounds they were too authoritarian, saw wealth, education, and liberty as self-reinforcing and in contrast to hunger, ignorance, and servitude. He viewed medicine as a social science and called politics "medicine on a grand scale." For an abridged version of his official report, see Virchow, Rudolf, "Report on the Typhus Epidemic in Upper Silesia", *American Journal of Public Health*, 2006, Vol. 96:12, pp. 2102-2105, http://www.ncbi.nlm.nih.gov/pmc/articles/PMC1698167/.

Bibliography

Alexander P.E. *et al.*, "World Health Organization recommendations are often strong based on low confidence in effect estimates", *Journal of Clinical Epidemiology,* 2014, Vol. 67:6, pp. 629-634, http://www.ncbi.nlm.nih.gov/pubmed/24388966 DOI: 10.1016/j/clinepi.2013.09.020.

Allsop K.A. and Brand Miller J., "Honey revisited: a reappraisal of hone in pre-industrial diets", *British Journal of Nutrition,* 1996, Vol. 75, pp. 513-520, http://www.ncbi.nlm.nih.gov/pubmed/8672404.

Anomaly J., "Is Obesity a Public Health Problem?", *Public Health Ethics,* 2012, Vol. 5:3, pp. 216-221, DOI: 10.1093/phe/phs028 35.

Atkins P.J., "The material histories of food quality and composition", *Endeavour,* 2011, Vol. 2-3, http://www.ncbi.nlm.nih.gov/pubmed/21924495.

Baillie-Hamilton P.F., "Chemical Toxins: A Hypothesis to Explain the Global Obesity Epidemic", *The Journal of Alternative and Complementary Medicine,* 2002, Vol. 8:2, pp. 185-192, http://encognitive.com/files/Chemical%20Toxins--%20A%20Hypothesis%20to%20Explain%20the%20Global%20Obesity%20Epidemic.pdf.

Barrowman N., "Correlation, Causation and Confusion", *The New Atlantis,* 2014, Vol. 43, pp. 23-44, http://www.thenewatlantis.com/publications/correlation-causation-and-confusion.

Blasbalg T.L. *et al.*, "Changes in consumption of omega-3 and omega-6 fatty acids in the United States during the 20th century", *American Journal of Clinical Nutrition,* 2011, Vol. 93:5, pp. 950-962, http://ajcn.nutrition.org/content/93/5/950.full DOI: 10.3945/ajcn.110.006643.

Blaser M.J. and Falkaw S., "What are the consequences of the disappearing human microbiota?", *Nature Reviews Micriobiology*, 2009, Vol. 7, pp. 887-894, http://www.nature.com/nrmicro/journal/v7/n12/full/nrmicro2245.html DOI: 10.1038/nrmicro2245.

Boonstra R., "Reality as the leading cause of stress: rethinking the impact of chronic stress in nature", *Functional Ecology*, 2013, Vol. 27:1, pp. 11-23, http://onlinelibrary.wiley.com/doi/10.1111/1365-2435.12008/full DOI:10..1111/1365-2435.12008.

Brandes E.W. and Sartoris G.B., "Sugarcane: Its Origin and Impovement", *Yearbook of the U.S. Department of Agriculture*, 1936, pp. 561-624, http://naldc.nal.usda.gov/naldc/download.xhtml?id=IND43893527&content=PDF.

Burgio E. *et al.*, "Obesity and diabetes: from genetics to epigenetics", *Molecular Biology Reports*, 2015, Vol. 42:4, pp. 799-818, http://www.ncbi.nlm.nih.gov/pubmed/25253098 DOI: 10.1007/s11033-014-3751-z.

Campos P. *et al.*, "The epidemiology of overweight and obesity: public health crisis or moral panic?", *International Journal of Epidemiology*, 2006, Vol. 6:35, pp. 55-60, http://ije.oxfordjournals.org/content/35/1/55.full DOI: 10.1093/ije/dyi254.

Campos P., "Food policy and cognitive bias", *Wake Forest Journal of Law & Policy*, 2015, Vol. 5:1, pp. 187-192, http://lawpolicyjournal.law.wfu.edu/files/2015/03/7-Campos_Final.pdf.

Clayton P. and Rowbotham J., "An unsuitable and degraded diet? Part one: Public health lessons from the mid-Victorian working class diet", *Journal of the Royal Society of Medicine*, 2008, Vol. 101:6, pp. 282-289, http://www.ncbi.nlm.nih.gov/pmc/articles/PMC2408622/ DOI: 10.1258/jrsm.2008.080112 [three-part series].

Cordain L. *et al.*, "Origins and evolution of the Western diet: health implications for the 21st century", *American Journal of Clinical Nutrition*, 2005, Vol. 81:2, pp. 341-354, http://ajcn.nutrition.org/content/81/2/341.full.

Creel S. *et al.*, "The ecology of stress: effects of the social environment", *Functional Ecology*, 2013, Vol. 27:1, pp. 66-80, DOI: 10.1111//j.1365-2435.2012/02029.x.

Davis C., "Results of the Self-Selection of Diets By Young Children", *Canadian Medical Association Journal*, 1939, Vol. 41:3, pp.257-261, http://www.ncbi.nlm.nih.gov/pmc/articles/PMC537465/.

Davis D.R. *et al.*, "Changes in USDA Food Composition Data for 43 Garden Crops, 1950 to 1999", *American College of Nutrition Journal*, 2004, Vol. 23:6, pp. 669-682, http://www.ncbi.nlm.nih.gov/pubmed/15637215.

Dobson A., "Food-web structure and ecosystem services; insights from the Serengeti", *Philosophical Transactions of the Royal Society B*, 2009, Vol. 364, pp. 1665-1682, http://rstb.royalsocietypublishing.org/content/royptb/364/1524/1665.full DOI: 10.1098/rstb.2008.0287.

Drewnowski A., "The Real Contribution of Added Sugars and Fats to Obesity", *Epidemiology Review*, 2007, Vol. 29:1, pp. 160-171, http://epirev.oxfordjournals.org/content/29/1/160.full DOI: 10.1093/epirev/mxm011.

Eknoyan G., "A History of Obesity, or How What Was Good Became Ugly and Then Bad", *Advances in Chronic Kidney Disease*, 2006, Vol. 13:4, pp. 421-427.

Elliott J., "Flaws, Fallacies and Facts: Reviewing the Early History of the Lipid and Diet/Heart Hypotheses", *Food and Nutrition Sciences*, 2014, Vol. 5, pp. 1886-1903, DOI: 10.4236/fns.2014.519201.

Elser J.L. *et al.*, "Regime Shift in Fertilizer Commoditie Indicates More Turbulence Ahead for Food Security", *Plos*, 2014, http colon /journals.plos.org/plosone/article?id=10.1371/journal.pone.0093998.

Ely J.J. *et al.*, "Diabetes and stress: an anthropological review for study of modernizing populations in the US-Mexico border region", *Rural and Remote Health*, 2011, Vol. 11:3, http://www.rrh.org.au/articles/subviewnew.asp?ArticleID=1758.

Englyst K.N. *et al.*, "Nutritional characterization and measurement of dietary carbohydrates", *European Journal of Clinical Nutrition*, 2007, Vol. 61, pp. 19-39, http://www.nature.com/ejcn/journal/v61/n1s/full/1602937a.html DOI:10.1038/sj.ejcn.1602937.

Ferrier P., "Food in popular literature", *Choices*, 2014, Vol. 29:1, http://www.choicesmagazine.org/choices-magazine/submitted-articles/food-in-popular-literature.

Fletcher A. *et al.*, "'We've Got Some Underground Business Selling Junk Food'. Qualitative Evidence of the Unintended Effects of English School Food Policies", *Sociology*, Vol 48:3, pp. 500-517, 2014. doi:10.1177/0038038513500102 or http://soc.sagepub.com/content/48/3/500.

Fraser D.W., "Vitamins and Vitriol: W.L. Braddon's Epidemiology of Beriberi", *American Journal of Epidemiology*, 1998, Vol. 148:6, pp. 519-527, http://aje.oxfordjournals.org/content/148/6/519.long.

Freedman D.H., "How Junk Food Can End Obesity: Demonizing processed food may be dooming many to obesity and disease", *The Atlantic*, July/August 2013, http://www.theatlantic.com/magazine/archive/2013/07/how-junk-food-can-end-obesity/309396/.

Genius S.J., "Pandemic of idiopathic multimorbidity", *Canadian Family Physician*, 2014, Vol. 60:6, pp. 511-514, http://www.cfp.ca/content/60/6/511.full.

Golubovic A., "Nutritional Advice Pertaining to Sugar in Post-WWII Canada", *M.A. thesis*, Dalhousie University, 2014, http://dalspace.library.dal.ca/handle/10222/54030?show=full.

Goryakin Y. *et al.*, "The impact of economic, political and social globalization on overweight and obesity in the 56 low and middle income countries", *Social Science & Medicine*, 2015, Vol. 133, pp. 67-76, http://www.ncbi.nlm.nih.gov/pmc/articles/PMC4416723/ DOI:10.1016/j.socscimed.2015.03.030.

Gracey M., "Historical, cultural, political, and social influences on dietary patterns and nutrition in Australian Aboriginal children", *American Journal of Clinical Nutrition*, 2000, Vol. 72:5, pp. 1361-1367, http://ajcn.nutrition.org/content/72/5/1361s.long.

Greenhalgh T., "Evidence based medicine: a movement in crisis?", *BMJ*, 2014, Vol. 348, http://www.bmj.com/content/348/bmj.g3725 DOI: 10.1136/bmj.g3725.

Griggs P., "A 'Natural Part of Life': The Australian Sugar Industry's Campaign to Reverse Declining Australian Sugar Consumption, 1980-1995", *Journal of Australian Studies*, 2009, Vol. 30, pp. 141-154, http://www.tandfonline.com/doi/abs/10.1080/14443050609388057#.VeDp6fmqqko DOI:10.1080/14443050609388057.

Gross L.S. *et al.*, "Increased consumption of refined carbohydrates and the epidemic of type 2 diabetes in the United States: an ecologic assessment", *American Journal of Clinical Nutrition*, 2004, Vol. 79:5, pp. 774-779, http://ajcn.nutrition.org/content/79/5/774.full.

Hacking I., "Kinds of People: Moving Targets", *British Academy Lecture 2006. Proceedings of the British Academy*, 2007, Vol. 151, pp. 285-318, DOI:10.5871/bacad/9780197264249.003.0010.

Hardin-Fanning F., "Adherence to a Mediterranean diet in a rural Appalachian food desert", *Rural and Remote Health*, 2013, Vol. 13, http://www.rrh.org.au/articles/subviewnew.asp?ArticleID=2293.

Harvill E.T., "Cultivating Our 'Frienemies': Viewing Immunity as Microbiome Management", *mBio*, 2013, Vol. 4:2, http://mbio.asm.org/content/4/2/e00027-13.full DOI: 10.1128/mBio.00027.

Hendrickx K., *Bodies of Evidence: An Anthropology of the Health Claim*, PhD dissertation, 2014, University of Liege, Belgium. http://orbi.ulg.ac.be/handle/2268/168359.

Hollander G.M., "Re-naturalizing sugar: narratives of place, production and consumption", *Social & Cultural Geography*, 2003, Vol. 4:1, pp. 59-73, http://www.uky.edu/~tmute2/geography_methods/readingPDFs/hollander_re-naturalize-sugar.pdf.

Hulme M., "The conquering of climate: discourses of fear and their dissolution", 2008, *The Geographical Journal*, Vol. 174:1, pp. 5-16, DOI: 10.1111/j.1475-4959.2008.00266.x,

Ioannidis J.P.A. and Schoenfeld J.D., "Is everything we eat associated with cancer? A systematic cookbook review", *American Journal of Clinical Nutrition*, 2013, Vol. 97:1, pp. 127-134, http://ajcn.nutrition.org/content/97/1/127.long DOI: 10.3945/ajcn.112.047142.

James W.P.T. and Ralph A., "Should the national diet be altered to prevent coronary disease?", *Proceedings of the Nutrition Society*, 1988, Vol. 47, pp. 3-8.

Johnson R.J. *et al.*, "Potential role of sugar (fructose) in the epidemic of hypertension, obesity and the metabolic syndrome, diabetes, kidney disease, and cardiovascular disease", *American Journal of Clinical Nutrition*, 2007, Vol. 86:4, pp. 899-906, http://ajcn.nutrition.org/content/86/4/899.long

Khoury C.K. *et al.*, "Increasing homogeneity in global food supplies and the implications for food security", *PNAs*, 2014, Vol. 111:11, pp. 4001-4006, http://www.pnas.org/content/111/11/4001.full DOI:

Klimentidis Y.C., "Canaries in the coal mine: a cross-species analysis of the plurality of obesity epidemics", *Proceedings B*, 2011, Vol. 278, pp. 1626-1632, http://www.ncbi.nlm.nih.gov/pmc/articles/PMC3081766/ DOI: 10.1098/rspb.2010.1890.

Klurfeld D.M., "What Do Government Agencies consider in the Debate Over Added Sugars?", *Advances in Nutrition*, 2013, Vol. 4:2, pp.257-261, http://advances.nutrition.org/content/4/2/257.full DOI: 10.3945/an.112.003004.

Krause M., "The Ruralization of the World", *Public Culture*, 2013, Vol. 25:2, http://publicculture.org/articles/view/25/2/the-ruralization-of-the-world.

L'Abbé M.R. *et al.*, "Approaches to removing trans fats from the food supply in industrialized and developing countries", *European Journal of Clinical Nutrition*, 2009, Vol. 63, pp. 50-67, http://www.nature.com/ejcn/journal/v63/n2s/full/ejcn200914a.htm DOI:10.1038/ejcn.2009.14.

Landecker H., "Food as Exposure: Nutritional epigenist and the new metabolism", *Biosocieties*, 2011, Vol. 6:2, pp.167-194, DOI:10.1057/biosoc.2011.1.

Landecker H., "Metabolism, Reproduction, and the Aftermath of Categories", *LIFE (UN)LTD.*, 2013, Vol. 11:3, http://sfonline.barnard.edu/life-un-ltd-feminism-bioscience-race/metabolism-reproduction-and-the-aftermath-of-categories/.

Larsen L.T., *Is Prevention Better Than Cure? Public Health Policy and the Circular Structure of Learning*, Paper presented at the American Political Science Association Annual Meeting, 2010, http://papers.ssrn.com/sol3/papers.cfm?abstract_id=1642354.

Larsen M.H., "Nutritional advice from George Orwell: Exploring the social mechanisms behind the overconsumption of unhealthy foods by people with low socio-economic status", *Appetite*, 2015, Vol. 91, pp. 150-156, http://www.ncbi.nlm.nih.gov/pubmed/25865664 DOI: 10.1016/j.appet.2015.04.001.

Leach J.D., "Human Evolution, Nutritional Ecology and Prebiotics in Ancient Diet", *Bioscience Microflora,* 2006, Vol. 25:1, pp. 1-8, https://www.jstage.jst.go.jp/article/bifidus/25/1/25_1_1/_pdf.

Logan A.C. *et al.*, "Natural environments, ancestral diets, and microbial ecology: is there a modern 'paleo-deficit disorder?", Parts I and II, *Journal of Physiological Anthropology,* 2015, Vol. 34, http://www.jphysiolanthropol.com/content/34/1/1 DOI: 10.1186/s40101-015-0041-y.

Lucock M.D. and Martin C.E. , "Diet and Our Genetic Legacy in the Recent Anthropocene: A Darwinian Perspective to Nutritional Health", *Journal of Evidence-Based Complementary & Alternative Medicine,* 2014, Vol. 19:1, pp.68-83, http://chp.sagepub.com/content/19/1/68.long DOI: 10.1177/2156587213503345.

Lustig R.H., "Fructose: It's 'Alcohol Without the Buzz'", *Advances in Nutrition,* 2013, Vol. 4:2, pp. 226-235, http://advances.nutrition.org/content/4/2/226.full.pdf DOI:10.3945/an.112002998.

Lustig R.H. *et al.*, "Public health: The toxic truth about sugar", *Nature,* 2012, Vol. 482, pp. 27-29, http://www.nature.com/nature/journal/v482/n7383/full/482027a.html DOI:10. 1038/482027a.

Marlow M.L., "Government Overreach on Obesity Control", *Journal of American Physicians and Surgeons,* 2015, Vol. 20:1, pp. 12-14, http://www.jpands.org/vol20no1/marlow.pdf.

Marmot M.G., "Status Syndrome: A Challenge to Medicine", *JAMA,* 2006, Vol. 295:11, pp. 1304-1307, http://jama.jamanetwork.com/article.aspx?articleid=202520 DOI:10.1001/jama.295.11.1304.

McAllister E.J. *et al.*, "Ten Putative Contributors to the Obesity Epidemic", *Critical Reviews in Food Science and Nutrition,* 2009, Vol. 49:10, pp. 868-913, http://www.ncbi.nlm.nih.gov/pmc/articles/PMC2932668/ DOI: 10.1080/10408390903372599.

McGill A.T., "Causes of metabolic syndrome and obesity-related co-morbidities Part 1: A composite unifying theory review of human-specific co-adaptations to brain energy consumption", *Archives of Public Health,* 2014, Vol.72:1, http://www.ncbi.nlm.nih.gov/pmc/articles/PMC4335398/ DOI:10.1186/2049-3258-72-30.

Mello F.F.C., "Payback time for soil carbon and sugar-cane ethanol", *Nature Climate Change,* 2014, Vol. 4, pp. 605-609, DOI: 10.1038.nclimate2239.

Meloni M. and Testa G., "Scrutinizing the epigenetic revolution", *Biosocieties*, 2014, Vol. 9:4, pp. 431-456, http://www.ncbi.nlm.nih.gov/pmc/articles/PMC4255066/ DOI:10.1057/biosoc.2014.22.

Monaghan L.F. *et al.*, "Obesity Epidemic Entrepreneurs: Types, Practices and Interests", *Body and Society*, 2010, Vol. 16:2, pp. 37-71, DOI: 10.1177/1357034X10364769.

Moore J.W., "Cheap Food and Bad Climate", *Critical Historical Studies*, 2015, Vol. 2:1, pp. 1-42, http://www.researchgate.net/publication/276411125_Cheap_Food_and_Bad_Climate_From_Surplus_Value_to_Negative_Value_in_the_Capitalist_World-Ecology DOI:10.1086/681007.

Mosby I., "Administering Colonial Science: Nutrition Research and Human Biomedical Experimentation in Aboriginal Communities and Residential Schools, 1942-1952", *Histoire Sociale*, 2013, Vol. 46:91, pp. 144-172, http://www.fns.bc.ca/pdf/AdministeringSocialScience.mosby.pdf DOI: 10.1353/his.2013.0015.

Nerlich B., "'The post-antibiotic apocalypse' and the 'war on superbugs': catastrophe discourse in microbiology, its rhetorical form and political function", *Public Understanding of Science*, 2009, Vol. 18:5, pp. 5740-590, DOI: 10.1177/0973772507087974.

Oliveira N.M., *et al.*, "Evolutionary limits to cooperation in microbial communities", *PNAS*, 2014, Vol. 111:50, http://www.pnas.org/content/111/50/17941.full DOI: 10.1073/pnas.1412673111.

Oliver J.E., *Fat Politics: The Real Story Behind America's Obesity Epidemic*, 2006, Oxford University Press.

Oster R.T. *et al.*, "Cultural continuity, traditional Indigenous language, and diabetes in Alberta First Nations: a mixed methods study", *International Journal For Equity in Health*, 2014, Vol. 13, http://www.equityhealthj.com/content/13/1/92 DOI:10.1186/s12939-014-0092-4.

Phalkey Revati K. *et al.*, "Systematic review of current efforts to quantify the impacts of climate change on undernutrition", *PNAs*, 2015, www.pnas.org/cgi/doi/10.1073/pas.1409769112.

Powell B. *et al.*, "Improving diets with wild and cultivated biodiversity from across the landscape", *Food Security*, 2015, Vol. 7:3, pp.535-554, http://link.springer.com/article/10.1007%2Fs12571-015-0466-5.

Renner M., *Conservative Nutrition: The Industrial Food Supply and Its Critics, 1915-1985*, PhD thesis, University of California, Santa Cruz, 2012, http://escholarship.org/uc/item/6nk2s73b.

Schuldt J.P. and Pearson A.R., "Nutrient-centrism and perceived risk of chronic disease", *Journal of Health Pyschology*, 2015, Vol. 20:6, pp. 899-906 DOI: 10.1177/1359105315573446.

Scrinis G., "On the Ideology of Nutritionism", *Gastronomica*, 2008, Vol. 8:1, pp. 39-48, DOI: 10.1525/CFC.2008.8.1.39.

Semba R.D., "The Discovery of the Vitamins", *International Journal of Vitamin & Nutrition Research*, 2012, Vol. 82:5, pp. 310-315, http://www.ncbi.nlm.nih.gov/pubmed/23798048 DOI:10.1024/0300-9831/a000124.

Simopoulos A.P., "The Mediterranean Diet: What Is So Special about the Diet of Greece? The Scientific Evidence", *Journal of Nutrition*, 2001, Vol. 1:131, pp. 3065-3073, http://www.ncbi.nlm.nih.gov/pubmed/11694649.

Slavin J., "The challenges of nutrition policymaking", *Nutrition Journal*, 2015, Vol. 14, http://www.nutritionj.com/content/14/1/15 DOI: 10.1186/s12937-015-0001-8.

Slavin J. and Erickson J., "Total, Added, and Free Sugars: Are Restrictive Guidelines Science-Based or Achievable?", *Nutrients*, 2015, Vol. 7:5, pp. 2866-2878, http://www.mdpi.com/2072-6643/7/4/2866/htm.

Snowden F., *Naples in the Time of Cholera*, Cambridge University Press, 1995.

Snowden F., *Epidemics and Western Society Since 1600*, Yale University lecture series transcript http://gelaam.org/uploads/2/7/9/2/2792936/epidemics_and_western_society.pdf.

Spary E.C., *Feeding France: New Sciences of Food, 1760-1815*, Cambridge University Press, 2014

Szreter S., "Rapid economic growth and 'the four Ds' of Disruption, Deprivation, Disease and Death: public health lessons from 19th-century Britain for 21st century China?", *Tropical Medicine and International Health*, 1999, Vol. 4:2, pp. 146-152, http://www.ncbi.nlm.nih.gov/pubmed/10206269.

Taubes G., "The science of obesity: what do we really know about what makes us fat?", *BMJ*, 2013, Vol. 346, DOI:10.1136/bmj.f1050.

Taylor R. and Rieger A., "Rudolf Virchow on the typhus epidemic in Upper Silesia: an introduction and translation", *Sociology of Health & Illness*, 1984, Vol. 6:2, pp. 201-217, http://onlinelibrary.wiley.com/doi/10.1111/1467-9566.ep10778374/pdf.

Testa P., *Obesity as a knowledge problem: A political economy of the American diet*, Manuscript, 2013, http://www.sdaeonline.org/wp-content/uploads/2013/09/Testa-Obesity.pdf.

Thompson A., *"I AM COLD LUNCH": An Anthropological perspective on children's cultural identity and understanding of food through an ethnographic study of food and eating in public elementary schools*, B.A. thesis, Pacific University, 2007, http://commons.pacificu.edu/cassoc/3/.

Thorburn A.W. *et al.*, "Slowly digested and absorbed carbohydrate in traditional bushfoods: a protective factor against diabetes?", *American Journal of Clinical Nutrition*, 1987, Vol. 48, pp. 98-106, http://ajcn.nutrition.org/content/45/1/98.long.

Tsai F. and Coyle J., "The Microbiome and Obesity: Is Obesity Linked to Our Gut Flora?", *Current Gastroentology Reports*, 2009, Vol. 11:4, pp. 307-313, http://www.ncbi.nlm.nih.gov/pubmed/19615307.

Tuohy Kieran M. *et al.*, "Metabolism of Maillard reaction products by the human gut microbiota: implications for health", *Molecular Nutrition & Food Research*, 2006, Vol. 50:9, pp. 847-857, http://www.ncbi.nlm.nih.gov/pubmed/16671057 DOI:10.1002/mnfr.200500126.

Ventres W. and Gusoff G., "Poverty Blindness: Exploring the Diagnosis and Treatment of an Epidemic Condition", *Journal of Health Care for the Poor and Underserved*, 2014, Vol. 25:1, pp. 52-62, http://www.ncbi.nlm.nih.gov/pubmed/24509012 DOI:10.1353/hpu.2014.0025.

Vittecoq M. *et al.*, "Cancer: a missing link in ecosystem functioning?", *Trends in Ecology and Evolution*, 2013, Vol. 13:11, pp. 628-635, DOI: 10.1016/j/tree.2013.07.005.

Von Hertzen L. *et al.*, "Natural immunity: Biodiversity loss and inflammatory diseases are two global megatrends that might be related", *EMBO Reports*, 2011, Vol. 12:11, pp. 1089-1093, http://www.ncbi.nlm.nih.gov/pmc/articles/PMC3207110/.

Warner J. *et al.*, "Can Legislation Prevent Debauchery? Mother Gin and Public Health in 18th-Century England", *American Journal of Public Health,* 2001, Vol. 91:3, http://www.ncbi.nlm.nih.gov/pmc/articles/PMC1446560/.

Weaver C.M., *et al.*, "Processed foods: contributions to nutrition", Scientific Statement from the American Society for Nutrition, *American Journal of Clinical Nutrition,* 2014, Vol. 99, pp. 1525-1542, http://ajcn.nutrition.org/content/early/2014/04/23/ajcn.114.089284 DOI: 10.3945/ajcn.114.089284.

Weaver L.J. and Venkat Narayan K.M., "Reconsidering the history of type 2 diabetes in India: Emerging or re-emerging disease?", *The National Medical Journal of India,* 2008, Vol. 21:6, pp. 288-291, http://www.ncbi.nlm.nih.gov/pubmed/19691218.

Wells J.C.K., "Maternal capital and the metabolic ghetto: An evolutionary perspective on the transgenerational basis of health inequalities", *American Journal of Human Biology,* 2010, Vol. 22:1, pp.1-17, http://onlinelibrary.wiley.com/doi/10.1002/ajhb.20994/abstract DOI: 10.1002/ajhb.20994.

Wheelwright J., "Risky medicine", *Aeon,* 2014, http://aeon.co/magazine/health/is-preventive medicine-its-own-health-risk/.

Williams *Alan,* "One economist's view of social medicine", *Epidemiology and Community Health,* 1979, Vol.33, pp.3-7 http://jech.bmj.com/content/33/1/3.full.pdf.

Zhao L., "The gut microbiota and obesity: from correlation to causality", *Nature Reviews Microbiology,* 2013, Vol. 11, pp. 639-647, http://www.nature.com/nrmicro/journal/v11/n9/full/nrmicro3089.html DOI:10.1038/nrmicro3089.

Zhu Xin-Guang *et al.*, "What is the maximum efficiency with which photosynthesis can convert solar energy into biomass?", *Current Opinion in Biotechnology,* 2008, Vol. 19, pp. 153-159. DOI: 10.1016/j.copbio.2008.02.004 http://sippe.ac.cn/gh/2008%20Annual%20Report/Zhu%20X-G.pdf.

Zimmet P.Z., "Diabetes epidemiology as a tool to trigger diabetes research and care", *Diabetologia,* 1999, Vol. 42, pp. 499-518, http://www.ncbi.nlm.nih.gov/pubmed/10333041.